MW01156742

Principles and Management of Pediatric Foot and Ankle Deformities and Malformations

Principles and Management of Pediatric Foot and Ankle Deformities and Malformations

Vincent S. Mosca, MD

Professor of Orthopedics, University of Washington School of Medicine

Pediatric Orthopedic Surgeon
Chief, Foot and Ankle Service
Director, Pediatric Orthopedic Fellowship
Former Director, Department of Orthopedics
Seattle Children's Hospital
Seattle, Washington

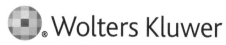

Wolters Kluwer
Health

Philadelphia • Baltimore • New York • London
Buenos Aires • Hong Kong • Sydney • Tokyo

Acquisitions Editor: Brian Brown
Production Development Editor: Dave Murphy
Production Project Manager: Priscilla Crater
Senior Manufacturing Manager: Beth Welsh
Marketing Manager: Daniel Dressler
Design Manager: Joan Wendt
Production Services: S4Carlisle Publishing Sevices

Two Commerce Square
2001 Market Street
Philadelphia, PA 19103 USA
LWW.com

Printed at Strategic Content Imaging

Library of Congress Cataloging-in-Publication Data

Principles and management of pediatric foot and ankle deformities and malformations / editor, Vincent S Mosca. — First edition
   p. ; cm.
Includes bibliographical references and index.
ISBN 978-1-4511-3045-4 (hardback : alk. paper)
I. Mosca, Vincent S., editor.
[DNLM: 1. Ankle—abnormalities. 2. Foot Deformities, Congenital—therapy. 3. Child. 4. Orthopedic Procedures—methods. WE 883]
RD563
617.5′85—dc23

                                                                                    2014010069

Care has been taken to confirm the accuracy of the information presented and to describe generally accepted practices. However, the authors, editors, and publisher are not responsible for errors or omissions or for any consequences from application of the information in this book and make no warranty, expressed or implied, with respect to the currency, completeness, or accuracy of the contents of the publication. Application of the information in a particular situation remains the professional responsibility of the practitioner.

The authors, editors, and publisher have exerted every effort to ensure that drug selection and dosage set forth in this text are in accordance with current recommendations and practice at the time of publication. However, in view of ongoing research, changes in government regulations, and the constant flow of information relating to drug therapy and drug reactions, the reader is urged to check the package insert for each drug for any change in indications and dosage and for added warnings and precautions. This is particularly important when the recommended agent is a new or infrequently employed drug.

Some drugs and medical devices presented in the publication have Food and Drug Administration (FDA) clearance for limited use in restricted research settings. It is the responsibility of the health care provider to ascertain the FDA status of each drug or device planned for use in their clinical practice.

To purchase additional copies of this book, call our customer service department at (800) 638-3030 or fax orders to (301) 223-2320. International customers should call (301) 223-2300.

Visit Lippincott Williams & Wilkins on the Internet: at LWW.com. Lippincott Williams & Wilkins customer service representatives are available from 8:30 am to 6 pm, EST.

Dedication

When asked in recent months how long it took me to write this book, I frequently replied "28 years," though the actual writing took 3 years of being glued to my computer most evenings and weekends. I now understand why most medical books are multiauthored.

I thank my beautiful wife and life partner, Shirley, for her patience, sacrifice, and support through this all-consuming process. We started our relationship not long before I started the writing phase. Having survived and thrived during this rigorous undertaking has great implications for our future together.

I am grateful to my lovely and talented daughter, Arianna, for sharing me with my demanding clinical and academic career during the last 18 years of the process, which were the first 18 years of her life.

Finally, I thank Dr. Lynn Staheli for 28 years of professional partnership, personal friendship, support, encouragement, mentorship, perspective, and role modeling. He showed me the way by word and by example.

Foreword

As a colleague, friend, and admirer, I have known Dr. Vincent Mosca for over 25 years. During this past quarter century, I have watched him evolve from a gifted, but inexperienced, pediatric orthopedic surgeon to his current status as the individual who many (including myself) consider to be the foremost international authority on foot deformities in children.

I attribute this evolution not only to Dr. Mosca's innate abilities as a clinician, surgeon, innovator, and teacher, but also to his willingness to focus his attention on the child's foot, an extensive, yet relatively neglected, field of study.

This book, Principles and Management of Pediatric Foot and Ankle Deformities and Malformations, is the culmination of Dr. Mosca's passion for the subject, his extensive experience and clinical research in the area, his innovations, and the honing of his ideas through decades of presentations to our resident staff as well as hundreds of invited lectures on the topic at national and international conferences. He has been awarded numerous University of Washington orthopedic teaching awards and is often sought as a faculty member for international seminars. In addition to his original research journal publications, he has written chapters on the child's foot in many of the major pediatric orthopedic textbooks.

In this book, Dr. Mosca correctly emphasizes the principles that prepare the reader to better understand the complexities of the child's foot. That understanding enables the serious reader to make the right clinical decisions regarding both simple and complex problems. This book provides the reader with the tools needed to understand and evaluate clinical problems and the detailed information required to manage them successfully while concurrently exposing the child to the least risk of complications.

Immediately obvious to the reader are the many full-color annotated illustrations and photos. The superb color photographs show Dr. Mosca's painstaking positioning of his camera for operative and clinical photographs. His operative images required hundreds of glove changes that allowed him to take the operative photographs himself from the bird's-eye view. This enabled him to show the pertinent anatomy clearly without the need for accompanying artist's sketches.

When these features are combined—a brilliant mind, years of experience, creativity, attention to detail, and a talent for teaching—this book is the outcome. Before reviewing the book, I predicted that the book would become a classic. After my review, I believe this prediction is confirmed and makes me believe that, for years to come, this book will be the foremost guide to the understanding and management of foot deformities in children.

Lynn T. Staheli, MD

Preface

"Techniques change, but principles are forever." The foot, and the child's foot in particular, is a complex anatomic body part with many bones, joints, muscles, and tendons working in concert to provide a stable, but supple, platform that helps it accommodate to the changing terrain below and propel the body in space. There are many congenital, developmental, and acquired deformities, as well as malformations, that challenge the ability of the foot to serve those complex and important functions. There is great variability in the natural history, severity, flexibility/rigidity, age at onset, age at treatment, and rate of progression of these conditions. Therefore, a principles-based approach is necessary to ensure the best possible treatment outcomes.

The traditional approach to treating foot deformities in children has been based on techniques. There is often a cookbook association of a named operation with a named deformity. However, there are many iatrogenic foot deformities and rare idiopathic deformities and malformations for which there are no reported cookbook treatments. Without a thorough understanding of foot deformities and malformations, it is challenging to determine what to do in these situations. Moreover, techniques change because of technologic advances and human creativity. Without a thorough understanding of foot deformities and malformations, it is difficult or impossible to assess and compare old and new techniques. The obvious conclusion is that the management of the varied, and often rare, foot deformities and malformations in children must be based on principles. And principles-based management is dependent on principles-based assessment.

A principle is a basic generalization that is accepted as true and can be used as a basis for reasoning or conduct. The purpose of this book is to present the principles of assessment and management of foot deformities and malformations in children and adolescents that have been conceived, developed, organized, and explained by one pediatric orthopedic surgeon with almost three decades of extensive experience studying and treating these conditions. The principles are then applied to the individual deformities and malformations. Finally, detailed descriptions of soft tissue and bony procedural techniques as performed by the author are presented, many of which are difficult or impossible to find elsewhere.

This book is not intended to be encyclopedic but, instead, practical and immediately applicable. Indications for nonoperative and operative management are stressed. Surgical techniques are described and illustrated. Pitfalls and complications of treatment are discussed.

How to use the book: Following the introductory chapter, **Chapters 2–4** elucidate the basic, assessment, and management principles needed to effectively treat foot deformities and malformations in children and adolescents. In **Chapters 5** and **6**, each of the major, and some of the minor, foot deformities and malformations is considered in regard to definition, elucidation of the segmental deformities, imaging, natural history, nonoperative treatment, operative indications, and operative treatment. The correction of most foot deformities and malformations involves the concurrent or sequential utilization of more than one soft tissue and/or bone procedure. To avoid redundancy, the procedures are individually described in detail in **Chapters 7** and **8**. The operative treatment section for each deformity and malformation in **Chapters 5** and **6** references the techniques in these final two chapters. The operative treatment section also indicates how the individual procedures are combined and, in some cases, modified for a particular condition.

This is a how-to book that is based on one surgeon's knowledge and extensive experience in this field. The principles are original to the author. The techniques are my originals or my interpretation/modification of the originals. The references at the end of the book allow the interested reader to access the original pertinent literature if, in fact, any exists.

I hope this book provides the reader with the knowledge and tools needed to meet the many challenges associated with the assessment and management of foot deformities and malformations in children.

Vincent S. Mosca, MD

Acknowledgments

I acknowledge my early "child's foot" teachers, in particular Drs. J. Leonard Goldner, Norris Carroll, and Colin Moseley, for their influences on my thought processes regarding deformities of the child's foot. Though I have come to different conclusions from theirs on how to manage some conditions, it is their reasoned, yet varied, approaches that led me to look for a way to resolve the discrepancies. My professional life's work has been devoted to resolving the discrepancies through the study and implementation of principles.

Table of Contents

CHAPTER *4*

CHAPTER 5

FOOT AND ANKLE DEFORMITIES 61

CHAPTER 6

FOOT MALFORMATIONS 119

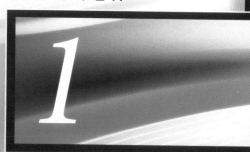
Introduction

"Techniques change, but principles are forever." I do not recall when I first heard that declaration or who in history first stated it, but it has been my mantra for decades. There may be no part of the human body for which the wisdom of those words is more poignant than the child's foot. With 26 bones, at least 31 articulations, and countless muscle/tendon attachments, the foot is comparable only to the hand as the most complex anatomic region of the musculoskeletal system. This anatomic complexity contributes to the extremely wide variety of deformities and malformations that afflict the foot. And although the incidence of malformations of the foot is comparable to that of the hand, there are far more deformations (deformities) of the foot than the hand.

PURPOSE OF THE BOOK

The foot, and the child's foot in particular, is a complex anatomic body part with many bones, joints, muscles, and tendons working in concert to provide a stable, but supple, platform that helps it accommodate to the changing terrain below and propel the body in space. There are many congenital, developmental, and acquired deformities, as well as malformations, that challenge the ability of the foot to serve those complex and important functions. There is great variability in the natural history, severity, flexibility/rigidity, age at onset, age at treatment, and rate of progression of these conditions. In addition, the effects of growth and development, as well as the effects of previous treatment, on the common and rare deformities and malformations of the child's foot make a cookbook approach to management unreasonable. That great variability also makes prospective, controlled studies of treatment effectiveness almost impossible to carry out. Therefore, a principles-based approach is necessary to ensure the best possible treatment outcomes.

The traditional approach to treating foot deformities in children has been based on techniques. There is often a cookbook association of a named operation with a named deformity. Unfortunately, the operation typically addresses only one or possibly two of the multiple deformities that are present. That approach can lead to poor surgical outcomes if the severity and rigidity of the deformities are greater than usual or if additional unrecognized segmental deformities exist. Furthermore, there are many iatrogenic foot deformities and rare idiopathic deformities and malformations for which there are no reported cookbook treatments. Without a thorough understanding of foot deformities and malformations, it is challenging to determine what to do in these situations. Moreover, techniques change because of technologic advances and human creativity. Without a thorough understanding of foot deformities and malformations, it is difficult or impossible to assess and compare old and new techniques. The obvious conclusion is that the management of the varied, and often rare, foot deformities and malformations in children must be based on principles. And principles-based management is dependent on principles-based assessment.

A principle is a basic generalization that is accepted as true and can be used as a basis for reasoning or conduct. The purpose of this book is to present, in one source, the principles of assessment and management of foot deformities and malformations in children and adolescents that have been conceived, developed, organized, and explained by one pediatric orthopedic surgeon with almost three decades of extensive experience studying and treating these conditions. The principles are then applied to the individual deformities and malformations. Finally, detailed descriptions of soft tissue and bony procedural techniques are presented, many of which are difficult or impossible to find elsewhere.

This book is not intended to be encyclopedic but, instead, practical and immediately applicable. Indications for nonoperative and operative management are stressed. Surgical techniques are described and illustrated. Pitfalls and complications of treatment are discussed.

For more detailed information on the definition, epidemiology, etiology, clinical features, radiographic features, pathoanatomy, natural history, and treatment of foot deformities and malformations in children, see my chapter entitled The foot. In: Weinstein SL, Flynn JM, eds. *Lovell and Winter's Pediatric Orthopedics*. 7th ed. Philadelphia, PA: Lippincott Williams & Wilkins; 2013:1425–1562. It is a valuable companion resource.

HOW TO USE THE BOOK

Following this introductory chapter, Chapters 2 to 4 elucidate the basic, assessment, and management principles needed to effectively treat foot deformities and malformations in children and adolescents. A thorough understanding of these principles is required before focusing on a particular foot deformity or malformation. In Chapters 5 and 6, each of the major, and some of the minor, foot deformities and malformations is considered in regard to definition, elucidation of the segmental deformities, imaging, natural history, nonoperative treatment, operative indications, and operative treatment. The correction of most foot deformities and malformations involves the concurrent or sequential utilization of more than one soft tissue and/or bone procedure. To avoid redundancy, the procedures are individually described in detail in Chapters 7 and 8. The operative treatment section for each deformity and malformation in Chapters 5 and 6 references the techniques in these final two chapters. The operative treatment section also indicates how the individual procedures are combined and, in some cases, modified for a particular condition.

The references are included at the end of the book, but are not annotated within the text. This is a "how to" book that is based on one surgeon's knowledge and extensive experience in this field. The principles are original to the author. The techniques are original to the author or the author's interpretation and/or modification of the originals. The references allow the interested reader to access the original pertinent literature.

Although the numerous images in this book should help clarify the principles and techniques for the reader, observation and manipulation of a life-size foot skeleton model (that is held together by elastic cords) will add three-dimensional clarity and should be used liberally.

To get started, definitions are in order.

Deformity/deformation: A *deformity/deformation* is a malalignment of relatively normally formed bones at a joint. A deformity can refer to malalignment at a single joint, but in most named deformities of the foot (clubfoot, cavovarus foot, skewfoot, etc.), there are at least two segmental deformities that are often in rotationally opposite directions from each other (**see Basic Principle #5, Chapter 2**). The malalignment may be (1) structural/rigid, i.e., characterized by restriction of normal joint motion, or (2) flexible, i.e., passively correctable. The latter may be idiopathic or dynamic (due to an underlying muscle imbalance). Structural/rigid and flexible deformities can be congenital, acquired, developmental, idiopathic, iatrogenic, caused by an underlying neuromuscular disorder, or some combination of these.

Malformation: A *malformation* is an incorrectly created anatomic part. Malformations fall into five broad categories: too large, too small, too many, too few, joined together/failed to separate (Table 1-1).

Congenital mal-deformation: Deformities can be associated with malformations. This is particularly true for malformations in the category of joined together/failed to separate and present at birth, i.e., congenital subtalar synostosis (**see Chapter 6**). In the flatfoot deformity associated with fibula hemimelia, Apert syndrome, and lower extremity hemiatrophy, there is congenital synostosis of the talus and calcaneus (and also commonly the cuboid and navicular). This is a failure of segmentation (failure of apoptosis) between the involved bones that begins as an extensive synchondrosis and undergoes metaplasia to a synostosis during early childhood. The calcaneus is attached to the talus in a laterally displaced position, creating valgus alignment of the hindfoot *without* the other components of eversion deformity of the subtalar joint. These rare, congenital, rigid flatfeet with extensive tarsal coalitions should perhaps be called *congenital mal-deformations*.

TABLE 1-1	Categories of Malformations

1. Too large
   a. Accessory navicular
   b. Longitudinal epiphyseal bracket
   c. Macrodactyly
   d. Gigantism
      i. Localized to forefoot
      ii. Total foot

2. Too small
   a. Brachydactyly
   b. Brachymetatarsia
   c. Hypoplasia

3. Too many
   a. Polydactyly

4. Too few
   a. Longitudinal deficiency
   b. Cleft foot (ectrodactyly)

5. Joined together (failed to separate)
   a. Syndactyly
      i. Simple
      ii. Complex
   b. Congenital synchondrosis/synostosis

Developmental mal-deformation: Congenital subtalar synostosis, a congenital mal-deformation, is quite different from the common, limited-size tarsal coalition. The latter is autosomal dominant, affects up to 13% of the population, and undergoes metaplasia from syndesmosis to synchondrosis to synostosis between the ages of 8 and 16 years, with progressive loss of subtalar motion and loss of longitudinal arch height (**see Chapter 5**). These are not congenital, though they are genetically programmed to develop. They result in a synostosis, which is a malformation, but not in the usual sense, in that they are not congenital, i.e., present at birth. Perhaps these should be called *developmental mal-deformations.*

Anatomic variation: And finally, one should be cautious in applying the term *deformity* to an *anatomic variation*. Most babies have physiologically normal, asymptomatic flexible flatfeet (**see Basic Principle #4, Chapter 2**). It is estimated that approximately 20% to 25% of adults have that same foot shape which, according to Harris and Beath, is the normal contour of a strong and stable foot and of little consequence as a cause of disability. Roughly 25% of the flatfooted adults, those with heel cord contractures, have pain (**see Chapter 5**). Perhaps, a painful flexible flatfoot with heel cord contracture should be called a deformity, and a painless flexible flatfoot without heel cord contracture should be considered merely an anatomic variation.

Though this classification system has never been formally proposed, I will refer to it from time to time in this book.

I hope this book provides the reader with the knowledge and tools needed to meet the many challenges associated with assessing and managing foot deformities and malformations in children.

Basic Principles

BASIC PRINCIPLE #1

Techniques change, but principles are forever.

Therefore, study principles! A principle is a basic generalization that is accepted as true and can be used as a basis for reasoning or conduct. There are many principles of assessment and management of foot deformities and malformations in children and adolescents that need to be appreciated and routinely utilized.

BASIC PRINCIPLE #2

A thorough knowledge of the normal anatomy of the child's foot is mandatory as the foundation for the assessment and management of foot deformities in children.

There are 26 bones and at least 19 major joints in a foot. The 52 bones in both feet represent 25% of all the bones in the body. Before treating deformities and malformations of the child's foot, whether nonoperatively or operatively, a thorough and working knowledge of the normal anatomy of the adult foot and ankle is required. Get a good anatomy book and study it. There are many available, but my favorite is *Sarrafian's Anatomy of the Foot and Ankle.* (See 3rd edition by Kelikian AS, editor. Philadelphia, PA: Lippincott Williams & Wilkins; 2011.) A thorough and working knowledge of the normal anatomy of the child's foot and ankle must then be acquired. Although all the same bones, joints, ligaments, muscles, and tendons are present in children and adults, the bones and joints are frequently aligned differently in the two age groups. To my knowledge, no anatomy book exists that is devoted exclusively to the normal child's

foot and its variations, so read on and you will learn what you need to know.

BASIC PRINCIPLE #3

The average normal foot shape in children is different than the average normal foot shape in adults.

And the range of normal foot shapes in children is different than the range of normal foot shapes in adults, though with significant overlap between age groups. For example, many or most babies are flatfooted, a shape less commonly seen in adults. Many babies have metatarsus adductus, a shape rarely seen in adults.

BASIC PRINCIPLE #4

Age-related anatomic variations in the shape of the foot and the natural history of each one must be appreciated.

This basic principle is a corollary of **Basic Principle #3**. In most cases, anatomic variations in the shape of the child's foot change spontaneously to adult norms through normal growth and development.

For example, most babies are flatfooted, whereas about 25% of adults are flatfooted (Figure 2-1). Approximately 1 in 100 babies have metatarsus adductus, almost none receive treatment, and very few adults have that foot shape (Figure 2-2).

Knowledge of anatomic variations and their natural history should prevent unnecessary and potentially harmful interventions.

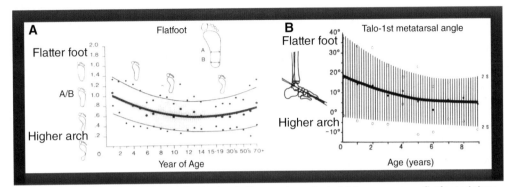

Figure 2-1. **A.** Footprints from individuals of all ages show that children are more flatfooted than adults, there is a wide range of normal arch heights, and the arch generally elevates spontaneously during the first decade of life. (From Staheli LT, Chew DE, Corbett M. The longitudinal arch. A survey of eight hundred and eighty two feet in normal children and adults. J Bone Joint Surg Am. 1987;69:426–428, with permission.) **B.** Radiographs from children of all ages confirm the footprint data. The drawing and graph represent the lateral talus–1st metatarsal (so-called Meary's) angle. (From Vanderwilde R, Staheli LT, Chew DE, et al. Measurements on radiographs of the foot in normal infants and children. J Bone Joint Surg Am. 1988;70:407–415, with permission.)

BASIC PRINCIPLE #5

"The foot is not a joint!" In all congenital and developmental deformities and most malformations of the child's foot, there are at least two segmental deformities that are often in rotationally opposite directions from each other, "as if the foot was wrung out" (Figure 2-3).

I conceived of, and published, these two phrases many years ago and continue to believe that they accurately and simply convey two important realities. Before one can surgically treat the pain and disability associated with foot deformities

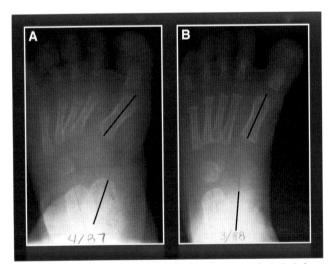

Figure 2-2. **A.** Anteroposterior (AP) radiograph of a baby's foot demonstrating forefoot adductus. (Some might argue that this is a skewfoot, though the strict differentiation of the two deformities in infancy has not been established.) **B.** AP radiograph of the same baby's foot 11 months later. The adductus has almost completely resolved without any treatment. NOTE: X-rays are not recommended to make or confirm the diagnosis of congenital metatarsus adductus in infants (**see Metatarsus Adductus, Chapter 5**).

and malformations, each segmental deformity and malformation must be identified, characterized, and understood so that a plan can be created to individually, yet concurrently, manage each one.

The rotationally opposite deformities are perhaps best appreciated in the cavovarus foot in which there are hindfoot varus and forefoot pronation, and the flatfoot in which there are hindfoot valgus and forefoot supination (Figure 2-3).

BASIC PRINCIPLE #6

One must understand subtalar joint positions and motions in a manner that supersedes the confusing and inconsistent terminology in the literature.

The static deformity positions of the subtalar joint can appropriately be described using the terminology used for other joints, i.e., varus (the calcaneus angles inward in relation to the talus) and valgus (the calcaneus angles outward in relation to the talus) (Figure 2-4).

Hindfoot varus is the static position of the subtalar joint found in cavovarus feet and clubfeet. Hindfoot valgus is the static position of the subtalar joint seen in flatfeet, skewfeet, and vertical tali. Some health care professionals use the term *pronated* when referring to a foot with hindfoot valgus. Forearms pronate and supinate. There is a lot more going on in foot deformities with a valgus hindfoot than can be captured with the simplistic and specific term *pronated* (**see Basic Principle #13, this chapter**).

The motions that result in those static positions should, in my opinion, be described using terms that recognize the unique and complex features of the subtalar joint. The subtalar joint differs from all other joints in the body in several ways: it is not a hinge joint or a ball-and-socket joint; its axis is not in the sagittal, coronal, or transverse plane; and it is a compound joint (several bones articulate) rather than a

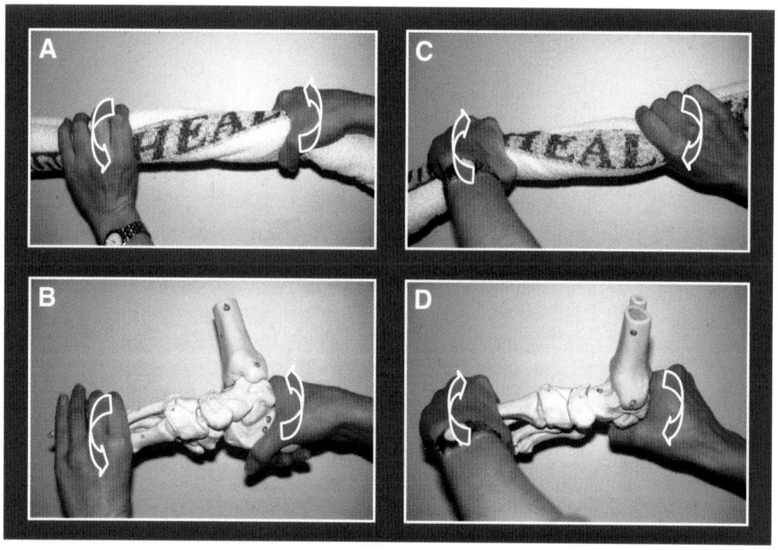

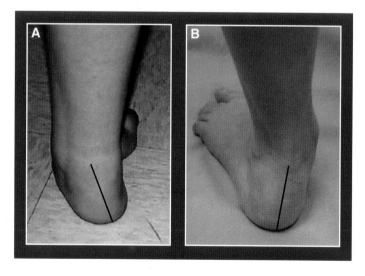

Figure 2-3. **A.** Towel wrung out. **B.** Foot model on elastic cords wrung out in the same manner, representing a cavovarus foot with hindfoot varus and forefoot pronation. **C.** Towel wrung out in the opposite direction. **D.** Foot model wrung out in the same manner, representing a flatfoot with hindfoot valgus and forefoot supination.

diarthrodial joint (two bones articulate). The subtalar joint complex is composed of 3 bones (possibly 4, if one includes the cuboid), several important ligaments, and multiple joint capsules that function together as a unit. Almost 200 years ago, Scarpa saw similarities between the hip joint and the subtalar joint complex. He coined the term *acetabulum pedis*, referring to a cup-like structure made up of the proximal articular surface of the navicular, the spring ligament, and the facets of the anterior end of the calcaneus (Figure 2-5).

He compared the femoral head to the talar head, and the pelvic acetabulum to his so-called acetabulum pedis (Figure 2-6).

I believe that the term *inversion* best captures the three-dimensional motions of the acetabulum pedis around the head of the talus that result in the static position "varus." The acetabulum pedis plantar flexes (down), internally rotates (in), and supinates. Simply stated, inversion is a "down and in" movement of the acetabulum pedis around the talus.

Conversely, *eversion* motion results in the static position "valgus." It is a combination of dorsiflexion (up), external rotation (out), and pronation of the acetabulum pedis around the talar head. Simply stated, eversion is an "up and out" movement of the acetabulum pedis around the talus (Figure 2-7).

BASIC PRINCIPLE #7

A thorough and working knowledge of the biomechanics of the foot, and of the subtalar joint complex in particular, is mandatory for assessment and management of foot deformities in children.

The functions of the foot include provision of a stable, but supple, platform that helps it accommodate to the changing terrain below and propel the body in space. And the subtalar joint is the machinery used by the foot to adapt to the

Figure 2-4. **A.** Hindfoot varus. **B.** Hindfoot valgus.

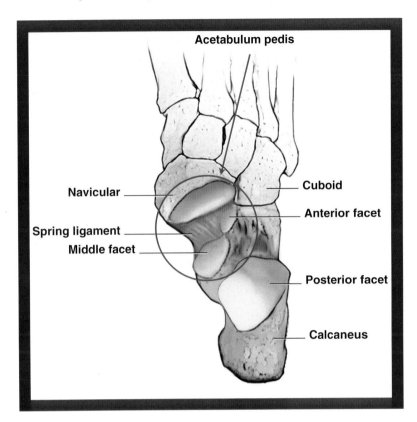

Figure 2-5. The acetabulum pedis, as conceptualized by Antonio Scarpa in 1818. It consists of the proximal articular surface of the navicular, the spring ligament, and the facets of the anterior end of the calcaneus.

ground during the early stance phase of gait and then convert to a rigid lever during push-off. Several authors have represented the complex interrelationships between the bones of the mid- and hindfoot as a mitered hinge, but that analogy is too simplistic. Using that as a first approximation or basic concept, one must add a thorough understanding of the shape, structure, relationships, and motions of the subtalar joint complex to truly understand the biomechanics of the foot.

As discussed in **Basic Principle #6**, Scarpa saw similarities between the hip joint and the subtalar joint complex and coined the term *acetabulum pedis*. Although it is not a perfect comparison, I believe that the two anatomic areas share certain features that make the comparison both valid and worthwhile. The hip, a pure ball-and-socket joint with a central point of rotation, is composed of 2 bones, 1 intraarticular ligament, and 1 joint capsule. The subtalar joint is not an independent ball-and-socket joint, though the

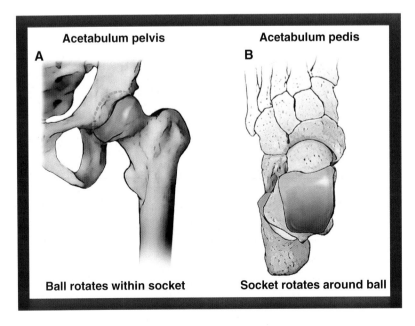

Figure 2-6. My concept of the comparison of the hip joint and the subtalar joint, as suggested by Scarpa. **A.** In the hip joint, the ball (the femoral head) rotates within the pelvic acetabulum. **B.** In the subtalar joint, the acetabulum pedis rotates around the ball (the talar head).

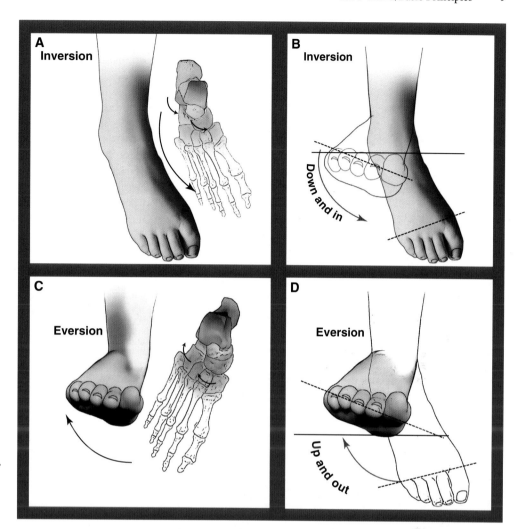

Figure 2-7. Subtalar joint motions. **A and B.** Inversion is plantar flexion, internal rotation, and supination of the acetabulum pedis around the talus—"down and in." **C and D.** Eversion is dorsiflexion, external rotation, and pronation of the acetabulum pedis around the talus—"up and out."

combined motions of the subtalar joint and the immediately adjacent ankle joint give the impression of a ball-and-socket. In fact, the subtalar joint has an axis of motion in an oblique plane that is neither frontal, nor sagittal, nor coronal

(Figure 2-8), thus creating motions that are best described by the terms *inversion* and *eversion* (Figure 2-7).

The stable structure in the hip joint is the acetabulum (the socket), while the stable structure in the subtalar joint

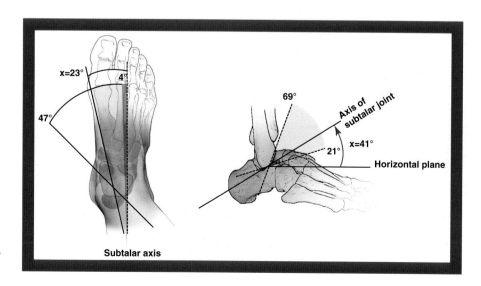

Figure 2-8. Axis of the subtalar joint.

complex is the talus (the ball). It is worth repeating that inversion comprises plantar flexion, internal rotation, and supination of the acetabulum pedis around the head of the talus—"down and in." Eversion is a combination of dorsiflexion, external rotation, and pronation of the acetabulum pedis around the talar head—"up and out." The static position of the inverted subtalar joint is called hindfoot varus, and the static position of the everted subtalar joint is called hindfoot valgus (Figures 2-4 and 2-7).

The tibia and talus internally rotate during the first half of the stance phase of the gait cycle while the subtalar joint complex everts. The acetabulum pedis dorsiflexes in relation to the talus, as a component of eversion. The foot becomes quite supple, or "unlocked," and the arch flattens. During the latter part of stance phase, the tibia and talus externally rotate while the subtalar joint complex inverts. The acetabulum pedis plantar flexes in relation to the talus, as a component of inversion, and once again supports the head of the talus. The subtalar joint and, thereby, the entire foot become rigid, or "locked" (Figure 2-9).

The foot acts as the most efficient and effective lever for the generation of power during push-off when the subtalar joint is inverted/locked and the foot is pointing directly forward, i.e., perpendicular to the transverse axis of the knee

joint. This is the concept of lever arm function. Lever arm dysfunction can result from shortening the lever arm and/or weakening the triceps surae. The lever arm is shortened when the foot is externally rotated in relation to the sagittal plane of the knee. This can be due to an everted/unlocked subtalar joint and/or external tibial torsion. The force coupling (force × distance to the center of the axis of motion, i.e., length of the lever arm) can be further diminished by weakness of the triceps surae. This can occur if the triceps surae is inappropriately lengthened and, thereby, weakened (Figure 2-10).

The ankle joint is also composed of three bones, several important ligaments, and one joint capsule. It is a hinge joint that functions strictly in the frontal plane. The talus plantar flexes (down) and dorsiflexes (up). It is important to reiterate, and to be constantly reminded, that the subtalar joint also plantar flexes and dorsiflexes, as components of the complex movements known as inversion ("*down* and in") and eversion ("*up* and out").

The talonavicular and calcaneocuboid joints are also known as Chopart joints and as the *transtarsal joints*. The talonavicular joint is the anterior extent of the subtalar joint complex and has the largest excursion of any part of it. The calcaneocuboid joint has only a toggle of motion, and on the basis of its position within the acetabulum pedis, one

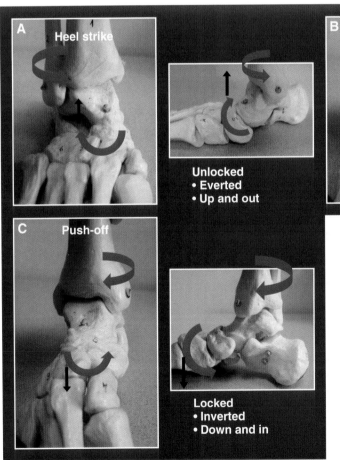
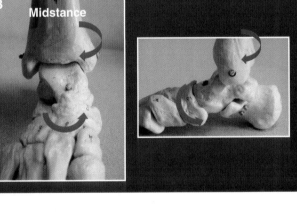

Figure 2-9. Unlocking and locking the subtalar joint during gait. **A.** At heel strike, the tibia/fibula/talus internally rotate as the subtalar joint everts ("up and out") (*purple curved arrows*). The acetabulum pedis dorsiflexes in relation to the talus (*black arrows*). The subtalar joint becomes supple, or "unlocked," in order to accept contact with the ground as the body's shock absorber. **B.** As stance phase progresses, the component parts reverse their rotation. **C.** At push-off, the tibia/fibula/talus are externally rotated and the subtalar joint is inverted ("down and in"), thereby plantar flexing the acetabulum pedis in relation to the talus (*black arrows*). The subtalar joint becomes "locked" so the foot can act as a rigid lever that is used by the triceps surae to generate power for push-off (**see Figure 2-10**).

Figure 2-10. **A.** Lever arm deficiency. Muscles always work as part of a force-couple (force × distance to the center of the axis of motion). Therefore, the plantar flexion/knee extension (PF/KE) couple depends on the appropriate alignment and rigidity of the foot. If this is not present, the extension moment against the knee will be inadequate even with adequate strength of the triceps surae. **B.** The black arrow shows a long lever arm in a foot with a neutral thigh–foot angle. External rotation of the foot shortens the lever arm (distance to the center of the axis of motion—*pink arrow*). The external rotation can be in the subtalar joint (as a component of eversion), or it can be due to external tibial torsion, or both.

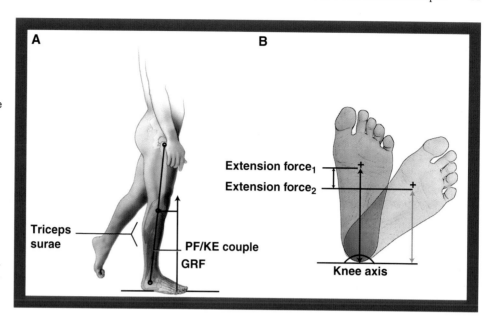

could consider it to be analogous to the transverse limb of the triradiate cartilage of the acetabulum of the hip joint (Figure 2-11).

The tarsometatarsal joints are also stable joints, with little more than a toggle of motion. The keystone architecture of the 2nd metatarsal–middle cuneiform joint helps to make it so. Hypermobility of the 1st metatarsal–medial cuneiform joint can cause painful pathology.

BASIC PRINCIPLE #8

In the normal foot, the overall shape is determined by the shapes and interrelationships of the bones, coupled with the strength and flexibility of the ligaments. Muscles maintain balance, accommodate the foot to uneven terrain, protect the ligaments from unusual stresses, and propel the body forward.

Basmajian performed electromyographic assessment of the muscles of the foot and ankle and showed little or no muscular activity when physiologic loads were applied to the static plantigrade foot. Muscular activity could be demonstrated only when very heavy loads were applied to the subjects. He concluded that the height of the longitudinal arch is determined by the bone–ligament complex and that the muscles maintain balance, accommodate the foot to uneven terrain, protect the ligaments from unusual stresses, and propel the body forward. Proponents of this bone–ligament

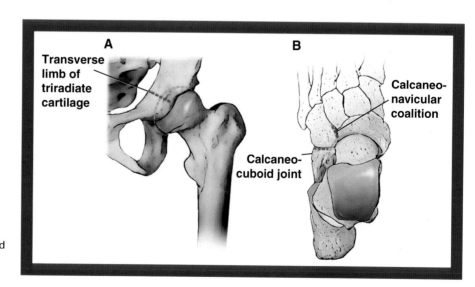

Figure 2-11. Considering Scarpa's analogy of the subtalar joint (**B**) to the hip joint (**A**), the calcaneocuboid joint is comparable to the transverse limb of the triradiate cartilage. Taking the analogy even further, a calcaneonavicular tarsal coalition might also be considered a type of transverse limb of the "triradiate cartilage" of the acetabulum pedis.

theory believe that the shape of the longitudinal arch under static loads is determined by the shapes and interrelationships of the bones, coupled with the strength and flexibility of the ligaments. Harris and Beath strongly supported this position and presented anatomic specimens to substantiate their theory. They were unable to determine whether the abnormal shapes of individual bones and joints represented a primary or secondary reflection of a long-standing flatfoot.

Most current authors conclude that excessive ligamentous laxity is the primary abnormality in flexible flatfoot (FFF) and that bone deformities are secondary. Muscles are necessary for function and balance, but not for structural integrity. Mann and Inman confirmed that muscle activity is not required to support the arch in static weight-bearing. They also found that the intrinsic muscles are the principal stabilizers of the foot during propulsion and that greater intrinsic muscle activity is required to stabilize the transverse tarsal and subtalar joints in a flatfooted individual than in one with an average-height arch.

BASIC PRINCIPLE #9

The default position of the subtalar joint is valgus/everted (Figure 2-12).

To my knowledge, this phenomenon has not been studied, but is due, in large part, to the shape of the subtalar joint facets and the alignment of the calcaneus under the talus. The midsagittal axis of the calcaneus is lateral to the midsagittal axis of the talus and the tibia (Figure 2-13).

The clinical importance and relevance of this phenomenon have to do with deformity correction surgery for cavovarus foot (varus hindfoot) and flatfoot (valgus hindfoot). Whereas medial soft tissue release is an important first step in correcting cavovarus deformity, lateral soft tissue release does nothing to correct flatfoot deformity (**see Management Principles #16 and 17, Chapter 4**).

BASIC PRINCIPLE #10

Valgus deformity of the hindfoot can be thought of as representing a continuum.

Here, I exclude consideration of the rigid flatfoot due to a tarsal coalition, since that is a developmental mal-deformation rather than a pure deformity. The etiologies and the natural histories of the pure valgus deformities are different, but valgus/eversion deformity of the hindfoot can be considered in relation to the severity of eversion, the flexibility of eversion, and the association with contracture of the tendo-Achilles. It ranges from mild, flexible physiologic to severe, stiff pathologic (Figure 2-14).

The natural history for the development of pain in FFF, flexible flatfoot with short Achilles (FFF-STA), and congenital vertical talus (CVT) is known. The natural history for the development of pain in congenital oblique talus (COT) has not been documented, because the very definition of the deformity is unknown. Therefore, the natural history must be assumed based on its position in the continuum of valgus deformity of the hindfoot (Figure 2-15).

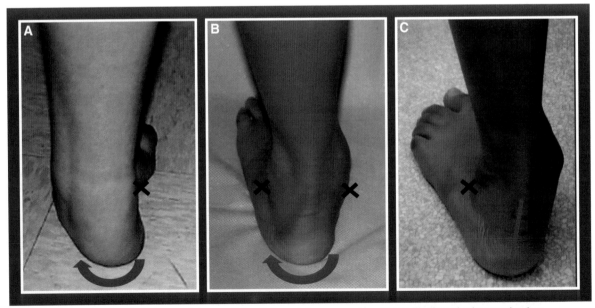

Figure 2-12. **A.** Release of the medial soft tissues in a cavovarus foot will allow the inverted subtalar joint to evert. **B.** In a neutrally aligned hindfoot, release of all of the ligaments around the subtalar joint will create eversion, i.e., a flatfoot. It will not invert. **C.** Release of the lateral soft tissues in a flatfoot will have no effect on the valgus/everted deformity.

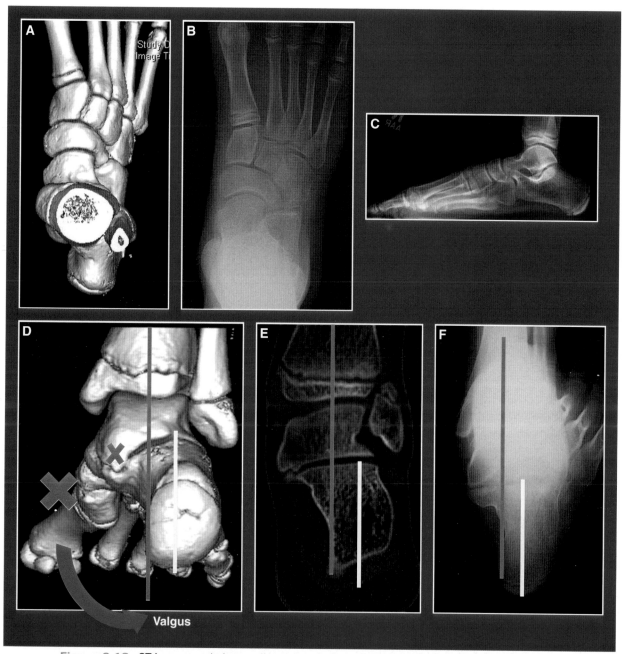

Figure 2-13. CT images and plane radiographs of a foot with average normal hindfoot alignment. It happens to have both calcaneonavicular (CN) and talocalcaneal (TC) tarsal coalitions, but shows normal hindfoot alignment very well, and so is being used to make a point. **A.** Dorsal view 3D CT reconstruction shows normal foot alignment. **B.** Standing AP radiograph shows normal foot alignment. **C.** Standing lateral radiograph shows normal foot alignment. **D.** Posterior view 3D CT reconstruction shows normal hindfoot alignment. The red line represents the midsagittal axis of the talus and the tibia, i.e., the axis of gravity. The yellow line represents the midsagittal axis of the calcaneus, which is lateral to the midsagittal axis of the talus and the tibia. Therefore, the subtalar joint will evert after a plantar–medial soft tissue release (*large red X*). It will also frequently evert after resection of a middle facet talocalcaneal tarsal coalition (*small red X*) if the subtalar joint is in valgus alignment before resection. **E.** Coronal slice CT image confirming comments made in **(D)**. **F.** Harris axial view plane radiograph confirming comments made in D.

Figure 2-14. One can reasonably consider valgus deformity of the hindfoot as a continuum. The etiologies and the natural history are different, but valgus/eversion deformity of the hindfoot ranges from the physiologic normal FFF (**A**) to the FFF-STA (**B**) to the COT (**C**) to the pathologic stiff CVT (**D**). This concept is helpful when considering the natural history of pain and dysfunction, particularly for the COT of which little is known.

BASIC PRINCIPLE #11

Cavus means hollow, empty, or excavated and is manifest in the foot by plantar flexion of the forefoot on the hindfoot. The plantar flexion may be along the medial column of the foot or across the entire midfoot. The subtalar joint may be in varus, neutral, or valgus. The ankle joint may be in plantar flexion (equinus), neutral, or dorsiflexion (calcaneus). And there may be a combination of these deformities (Figure 2-16).

Cavus deformity is shorthand for a quite varied group of deformities that share in common one feature; part or all of the forefoot is plantar flexed on the hindfoot, giving the appearance of a high arch.

BASIC PRINCIPLE #12

The foot deformity may be the primary problem or the result of the primary problem, i.e., a neuromuscular disorder. Differentiation is important (see Assessment Principle #3, Chapter 3).

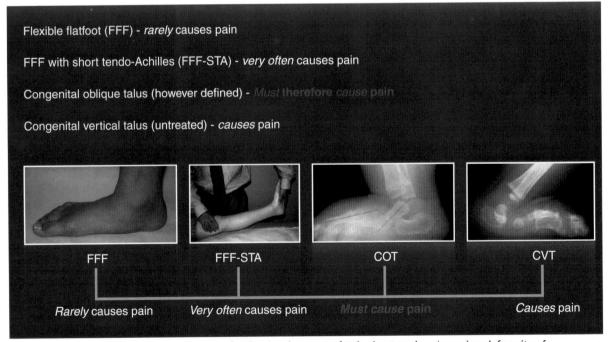

Figure 2-15. The natural history for the development of pain due to valgus/eversion deformity of the hindfoot is known for all except the COT, because so little is known about that condition in general. By considering COT in this proposed deformity continuum, one can assume its natural history to be that of the development of pain.

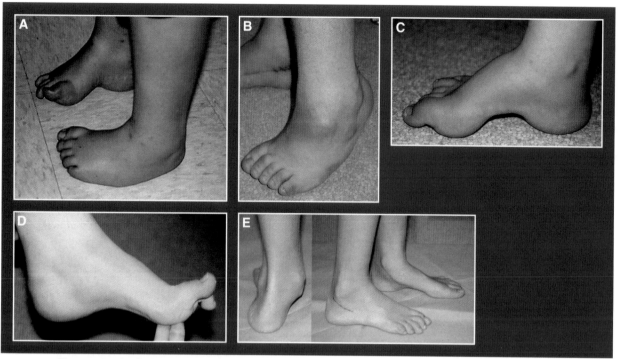

Figure 2-16. **A.** Cavovarus. **B.** Equinocavovarus. **C.** Calcaneocavus (a.k.a. transtarsal cavus). **D.** Equinocavus. **E.** Calcaneocavovalgus.

The apex of the longitudinal arch generally points in the direction of the primary problem (Figure 2-17).

In a cavus foot deformity, the apex of the arch is dorsal and points toward the muscles, nerves, spine, and brain. A cavovarus foot deformity is the result of a neuromuscular disorder until proven otherwise. It is important to remember this because a treatable neuromuscular disorder, such as a tethered spinal cord or spinal tumor, is not necessarily readily apparent when a child presents with a cavovarus foot deformity. However, it should be diagnosed and treated before the foot deformity is treated. Further permanent neuromuscular deterioration should be arrested as soon as possible. In a flatfoot, the apex of the longitudinal arch is plantar, essentially pointing to the foot itself. Flatfoot is most often either a normal anatomic variant or the primary problem. Examples of the latter include FFF-STA, tarsal coalition, CVT, and skewfoot. Flatfoot can also be associated with neuromuscular

disorders, such as cerebral palsy (CP), but these underlying disorders are usually apparent.

BASIC PRINCIPLE #13

Be accurate with terminology.

Do not use the term *pronated* as a substitute for the term *flatfoot*. There is very little pronation in a flatfoot, yet many health care professionals refer to a flatfoot as a pronated foot. It is true that pronation is one of the components of eversion of the subtalar joint, but the dorsiflexion and external rotation components are far more significant deformities. And the forefoot in a flatfoot is supinated! If it were not supinated, but instead followed the subtalar joint into eversion/"pronation," it might be appropriate to use the term *pronated*. In that situation, the lateral forefoot would be

Figure 2-17. **A.** In a flatfoot, the apex of the longitudinal arch is plantar, essentially pointing to the foot itself. A flatfoot is either normal or, if pathologic, it is usually the primary problem. **B.** In a cavus foot deformity, the apex of the arch is dorsal and points toward the muscles, nerves, spine, and brain, which are usually the underlying cause of the deformity.

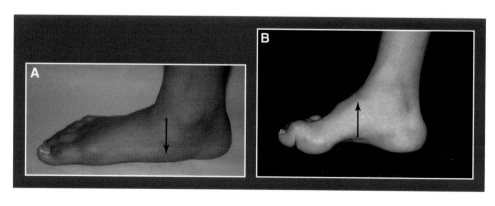

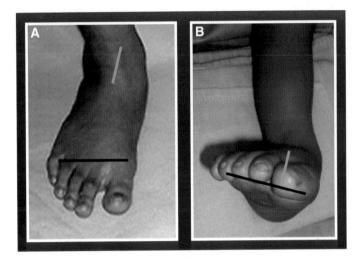

Figure 2-18. **A.** Physiologic FFF. The hindfoot is in valgus alignment in relation to the tibia (*green line*). The forefoot is supinated in relation to the hindfoot with all metatarsal heads on the ground (*black line*). **B.** Pronated foot in a child with fibula hemimelia and congenital subtalar synostosis. There is valgus alignment of the hindfoot in relation to the tibia (*green line*). The forefoot (*black line*) is in neutral rotation (neither supinated nor pronated) in relation to the hindfoot. The entire foot is pronated in relation to the tibia with the 5th metatarsal off the ground in weight-bearing.

elevated off the ground, a deformity that almost never exists except in some cases of congenital subtalar synostosis (**see Chapter 6**) (Figure 2-18).

Another misnomer for flatfoot that is often used when discussing adult flatfoot is "dorsolateral peritalar subluxation." It is true that eversion of the subtalar joint results in dorsal and lateral *positioning* of the navicular in relation to the head of the talus, i.e., peritalar. But there is no subluxation of any component part of the subtalar joint complex with even severe eversion. Subluxation means incomplete or partial dislocation of a joint, i.e., only partial contact between articular surfaces that normally have full contact. Dislocation means complete loss of contact between articular surfaces at a joint in which full contact normally exists.

Think of Scarpa's analogy of the hip and the acetabulum pedis (**see Basic Principles #6 and 7, this chapter**). Dorsolateral peritalar dislocations, like hip dislocations, can occur following severe trauma. There are also congenital hip dislocations and congenital talonavicular joint dislocations, the latter found in congenital vertical talus (CVT) deformities. Congenital and developmental (cerebral palsy, myelomeningocele, Down syndrome, Charcot-Marie-Tooth) hip subluxations occur, and these are characterized by partial contact (incongruity) between the femoral head and the acetabulum. There is no analogy for that pathology in the foot. Severe eversion, which might be called dorsolateral peritalar *positioning*, is a rotational malalignment of the subtalar joint that is perhaps analogous to severe abduction or adduction of the hip without translational loss of contact of the articular surfaces, i.e., without subluxation.

The term *flatfoot* has historical precedence and, though not specific, is associated with a good visual for most people. Use it. When describing isolated dorsolateral peritalar *positioning*, one can use that term or the terms *hindfoot valgus* or *hindfoot eversion*.

Cavus is defined as plantar flexion of the forefoot on the hindfoot. It does not mean "high arch," though that is the resultant effect. There may be plantar flexion of the medial column, the lateral column, or the entire forefoot on the hindfoot. The subtalar joint can be inverted, everted, or in neutral alignment. And the ankle can be plantar flexed, dorsiflexed, or in neutral alignment. When describing a cavus foot, it is best to describe all of its features. Some examples are cavovarus, equinocavovarus, calcaneocavus, and transtarsal cavus. I have seen congenital and iatrogenic calcaneoabducto-cavo-valgus (Figure 2-16).

BASIC PRINCIPLE #14

Do not focus entirely on the foot. There is an entire child above the foot.

It is important to remember this because management of clubfoot, for example, varies depending on whether it is an idiopathic deformity or one associated with myelomeningocele or arthrogryposis. Another example is intoeing in an older child with idiopathic clubfoot, which is usually due, at least in part, to femoral anteversion. Myopic focus on the foot is dangerous (**see Assessment Principles #2 and #7, Chapter 3**).

Assessment Principles

ASSESSMENT PRINCIPLE #1

A complete and detailed clinical and radiographic assessment of the child's foot is required before treatment is initiated.

It is hard to further clarify or justify this principle. How to do it is the focus of this chapter.

HISTORY

ASSESSMENT PRINCIPLE #2

Clinical evaluation of the child's foot begins with a clinical evaluation of the child.

Although the foot deformity or malformation is the reason for the requested evaluation by you, children with these conditions often have underlying neuromuscular, genetic, or chromosome disorders as well as other deformities and/or malformations of the lower extremities and spine. These must be recognized and factored into the decision-making process to ensure that the most appropriate of the possible nonoperative and operative interventions is chosen (**see Basic Principle #14, Chapter 2**).

Idiopathic congenital clubfoot, congenital vertical talus, flatfoot, metatarsus adductus, skewfoot, and positional calcaneovalgus deformity are often seen in normal children. These deformities can also be seen in children with underlying neuromuscular, genetic, or chromosome disorders. By way of contrast, almost all cavus foot deformities are the result of an underlying neuromuscular disorder, though congenital idiopathic cavus exists.

Foot deformities in children with neuromuscular, genetic, and chromosome disorders have appearances similar to those in normal children, but the natural history and response to treatment are often quite different. Therefore, differentiation is important.

Underlying conditions that are associated with congenital foot deformities and mal-deformations include myelomeningocele, lipomeningocele, arthrogryposis, sacral agenesis, fibular and tibial hemimelia, Apert syndrome, congenital hemiatrophy, myotonic dystrophy, Down syndrome, Ehlers–Danlos and Marfan syndromes, and a whole host of other chromosome abnormalities.

ASSESSMENT PRINCIPLE #3

Congenital and developmental deformities should be differentiated (*see Basic Principle #12, Chapter 2*).

Ask if the deformity was present at birth. Congenital deformities are rarely progressive in their natural history, yet rarely regressive. Tendons and joint capsules are usually co-contracted. For example, in a clubfoot (congenital talipes equinocavovarus) in an older child that does not correct with nonoperative management, posterior ankle capsulotomy is often required in addition to tendo-Achilles lengthening.

Developmental deformities, by definition, are progressive in their natural history, though the rate of progression is variable. Contracture of tendons precedes contracture of joint capsules. In a developmental equinocavovarus foot deformity in an older child, an tendo-Achilles lengthening is usually sufficient to correct the equinus deformity.

ASSESSMENT PRINCIPLE #4

Static and progressive foot deformities should be differentiated, and the rate of progression established, if possible.

Ask if the deformity has changed noticeably over time and, if so, by how much over what interval. As stated in **Assessment Principle #3**, most congenital foot deformities are static, rather than progressive, in nature. Muscle imbalance is the underlying problem in many acquired foot deformities. The muscle imbalance can be static, as in children with myelomeningocele, lipomeningocele, and postinfectious poliomyelitis; or it can be progressive, as in children with Charcot–Marie–Tooth disease, muscular dystrophy, spinal cord tumors, tethered cord, and diastematomyelia. Whether the muscle imbalance is static or progressive, the deformity is likely to progress. Unfortunately, the rate of progression is rarely predictable for either static or progressive muscle imbalances. Progression will increase the complexity of reconstruction.

ASSESSMENT PRINCIPLE #5

It is often more challenging to ascertain the history of pain and/or dysfunction that is related to a foot deformity in a child than in an adult, but it is worth the effort.

Otherwise, it is like practicing veterinary medicine. Reasons for children to be poor historians include too young, "too adolescent," intellectually challenged, neurologically impaired. The importance of an accurate assessment of the pain and dysfunction is that there are many clinically and radiographically apparent normal anatomic variations of the child's foot. If the pain location, severity, and temporal and activity-related patterns do not match the known pain pattern of a particular deformity/condition, the two might not be related. Do not go for the low-hanging fruit.

ASSESSMENT PRINCIPLE #6

Assessment of pain must be specific—ask where, when, what level/severity, what associations.

There are many anatomic variations of the foot, including a host of accessory ossicles, which could be the source of pain or merely incidental findings. It is easy, for example, to ascribe reported foot pain to a tarsal coalition or an accessory navicular that is identified on an x-ray. However, since most anatomic variations including tarsal coalitions and accessory naviculars do not hurt, it is important to know the exact site(s) of pain (**see Assessment Principle #15, this chapter**), as well as the activities that incite and relieve the pain. Severity of the pain should be quantified. Visual analog pain scales have been shown to be reliable in even very young children. The pain location, pattern, and severity must all match those of the presumed diagnosis. Chronic pain in a nonphysiologic distribution that occurs continuously during all waking hours and is reported to be of an exaggerated severity suggests chronic regional pain syndrome, a.k.a. reflex sympathetic dystrophy, reflex neurovascular dystrophy, and pain amplification syndrome.

PHYSICAL EXAMINATION

ASSESSMENT PRINCIPLE #7

Physical evaluation of the child's foot begins with a physical evaluation of the child (*see Basic Principle #14, Chapter 2*).

This includes a careful examination of the hips and spine in a newborn. Visual gait analysis, torsional profile analysis, and angular alignment assessment are used for older children and adolescents.

Visual gait analysis is carried out by watching the child walk, run, toe walk, heel walk, squat and stand, and hop on each foot. These observations are used to evaluate symmetry, strength, coordination, and comfort.

The child's torsional profile must be ascertained. The foot progression angle, which is assessed while the child walks at a normal pace in a long hallway, is the summation of all segmental rotational alignments/deformities in the lower extremities. The segmental rotational alignment values are determined with the child prone on an examination table. The degrees of internal and external hip rotation reflect femoral torsion. Utilization of the thigh–foot angle (TFA) for assessment of tibial torsion is predicated on the absence of a foot deformity in the limb being tested. Determination of the transmalleolar axis (TMA) is required to assess tibial torsion when there is hindfoot/subtalar joint deformity and/or equinus deformity. Assessment of the TMA is less reliable than assessment of the TFA.

The importance of accurate assessment of lower limb torsion is highlighted in children with flatfoot deformity, whether idiopathic or associated with cerebral palsy or tarsal coalition. There is rarely coincident pathologic tibial torsion in these conditions. The external rotation of the foot in relation to the limb exists almost entirely in the subtalar joint. A flatfoot will create an out-turned, or positive value, TFA because of eversion/external rotation of the subtalar joint (up and *out*) (**see Basic Principles #6 and 7, Chapter 2**). If the clinical TFA equals the radiographic standing anteroposterior (AP) talus–1st metatarsal (MT) angle (**see Assessment Principle #18, this chapter**). All of the external rotation is in the subtalar joint (foot) and none in the tibia. If the TFA is greater than the standing AP talus–1st MT angle, the difference is the degree of external tibial torsion.

In contrast, developmental cavovarus foot deformities are usually associated with external tibial torsion which is exposed after the foot deformity is corrected. A cavovarus deformity will internally rotate the foot in relation to the limb because of inversion/internal rotation of the subtalar joint (down and *in*) (**see Basic Principles #6 and 7, Chapter 2**). The thigh–foot angle is neutral to slightly internally rotated before the foot surgery and outwardly rotated afterward, reflecting the external tibial torsion that was already present. Families need to be apprised of this fact before the foot surgery is performed, or they will assume that the foot deformity was overcorrected (**see Management Principle #10, Chapter 4**). The change in TFA after correction of a cavovarus deformity will equal the preoperative AP talus–1st MT angle (**see Assessment Principle #18, this chapter**).

Equinus deformity will also make it challenging to determine tibial torsion using the TFA, because the planar axis of the foot is not parallel with the planar axis of the femur. The TMA is necessary to determine tibial torsion in this situation as well.

TABLE 3-1

Deformity-specific segmented deformities of the foot and ankle

	Forefoot	Midfoot	Hindfoot	Ankle
Clubfoot	Pronated	Adducted	Varus/inverted	Plantar flexed
Cavovarus	Pronated	Adducted or neutral	Varus/inverted	Plantar flexed, neutral, or dorsiflexed
Flatfoot	Supinated	Abducted or neutral	Valgus/everted	Plantar flexed
Vertical talus	Supinated	Abducted or neutral, dorsally dislocated	Valgus/everted	Plantar flexed
Met adductus	Neutral or supinated	Adducted	Neutral	Neutral
Skewfoot	Pronated, plantar flexed	Adducted	Valgus/everted	Plantar flexed or neutral

Exaggerated genu varum and genu valgum will cause the foot to bear weight unusually because of the altered angular relationship between the tibia and the ground. This can create an apparent foot deformity when none exists.

ASSESSMENT PRINCIPLE #8

Assessment of each of the segmental deformities of the foot and ankle is imperative before planning treatment, as a plan needs to be established to correct each one (*Table 3-1, Figure 3-1*).

The segments are:
1. Forefoot—pronated or supinated; plantar flexed (equinus) or dorsiflexed
   a. Recall that alignment (and deformity) is defined as the relationship between a more distal anatomic part and the next more proximal anatomic part. Therefore, pronation or supination refers to the alignment of the forefoot in relation to the midfoot/hindfoot, not the tibia/leg. This has been a source of confusion for many who believe the forefoot in a flatfoot is neutrally aligned (in relation to the tibia) when, in fact, it is supinated—in relation to the mid/hindfoot (*Figure 3-2*).
2. Midfoot—abducted or adducted (**see Metatarsus adductus, Chapter 5**)
3. Hindfoot—varus/inverted or valgus/everted (**see Figures 2-4 and 2-7, Chapter 2**)

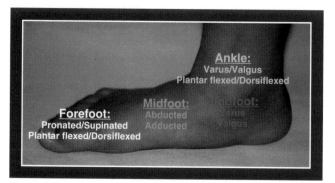

Figure 3-1. Identify each of the segmental deformities of the foot and ankle before initiating treatment.

4. Ankle—varus or valgus (**see Figure 3-12, this chapter**); plantar flexed (equinus) or dorsiflexed (calcaneus)

ASSESSMENT PRINCIPLE #9

Each segment of the foot should be evaluated for shape/deformity, flexibility, and skin integrity. Documentation should be specific.

Accurate assessment of the shape of each segment of the foot is the first step. For a cavovarus foot deformity, the segmental deformities are pronation of the forefoot, adduction of the midfoot, varus of the hindfoot, and possibly equinus of the ankle (Table 3-1). Equally important is the flexibility of each segment. The first segment to lose flexibility is the forefoot. Loss of flexibility of the hindfoot, which is assessed by the Coleman block test, eventually follows (Figure 3-3).

I have found that the block test, as described by Coleman, is uncomfortable and awkward to perform and, therefore, unreliable. With the entire lateral column of the foot on the block, it is tempting for the child to balance the foot on the block, rather than allowing the forefoot to pronate off the block. Price and Mubarak have independently proposed alternate methods for the clinical assessment of hindfoot flexibility in a cavovarus foot. However, neither is performed in weight-bearing. A more comfortable, reliable, and accurate way to assess weight-bearing hindfoot flexibility in a cavovarus foot is to perform a modified Coleman block test in which a 2.5-cm block is placed under the lateral 2–3 MT heads. The heel remains on the ground and the medial MT heads seek the ground as the forefoot pronates off the block (Figure 3-4).

Skin integrity should be assessed, as it can identify unsafe foot pressures which is especially important in children with insensate skin. In the cavovarus foot, exaggerated pressures are seen at the base of the 5th MT and under the 1st and 5th MT heads (Figure 3-5).

The segmental deformities of a flatfoot include supination of the forefoot, abduction or straight alignment of the midfoot, valgus of the hindfoot, and equinus of the ankle (Table 3-1). Equally important is the flexibility of each segment. Flexibility of the hindfoot is assessed in a different

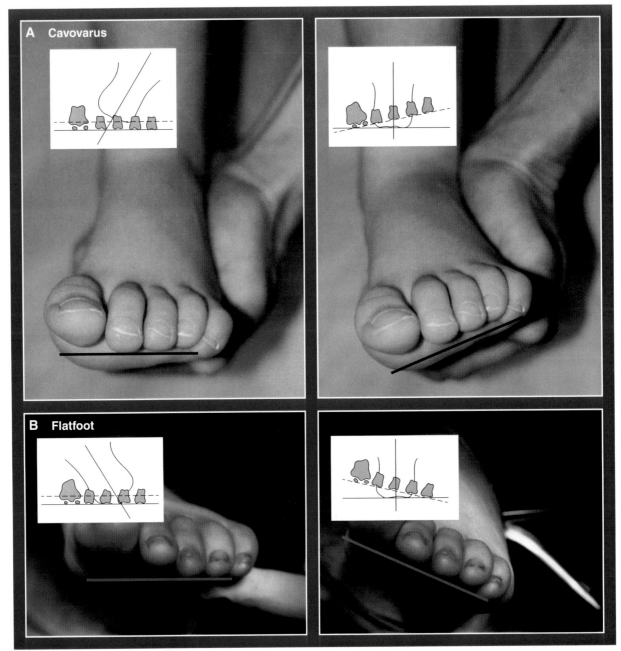

Figure 3-2. **A.** Pronation of the forefoot in a cavovarus foot is unappreciated until the hindfoot varus is corrected to neutral. **B.** Supination of the forefoot in a flatfoot is unappreciated until the hindfoot valgus is corrected to neutral.

manner than that used for a cavovarus foot. There is not a reliable "reverse" Coleman block test. Instead, toe standing (Figure 3-6) and the Jack toe raise test are utilized to assess hindfoot flexibility (Figure 3-7).

Evidence of exaggerated skin pressures in a flatfoot are identified under the medial midfoot. The skin in this area is rarely stressed except when a flatfoot is associated with contracture of the gastrocnemius or the entire triceps surae (tendo-Achilles) (Figure 3-8).

The clubfoot should be assessed for shape and flexibility using one or both of the two most commonly used classification systems, those of Pirani and Dimeglio.

ASSESSMENT PRINCIPLE #10

The accurate assessment of subtalar motion is an inexact science, but you can better at it by practicing.

There are no studies documenting the accuracy of assessment of subtalar motion. It is particularly challenging in very small feet and fat feet. The ankle should be held in neutral dorsiflexion. The dome of the talus is biconical in shape, narrower posteriorly than anteriorly. Dorsiflexion of the foot engages the widest portion of the talar dome in the ankle mortis, thereby creating bony stability as well as tightening

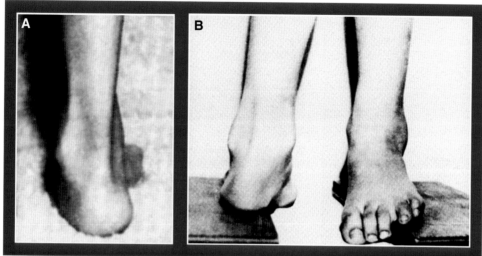

Figure 3-3. The Colman block test is used to assess flexibility of the hindfoot in a cavovarus foot with rigid forefoot pronation. Early in the course of development of the cavovarus deformity, the hindfoot varus (seen in **A**) remains flexible despite rigid forefoot pronation. It corrects to valgus (seen in **B**) with a block of wood under the lateral forefoot which allows the forefoot to pronate freely over the edge of the block. At that stage, correction of the forefoot deformity alone will result in spontaneous correction of the hindfoot. In time, the hindfoot varus deformity becomes rigid. Correction of the hindfoot deformity must then be combined with correction of the forefoot deformity. (From Coleman SS, Chestnut WJ. A simple test for hindfoot flexibility in the cavovarus foot. Clin Orthop Relat Res. 1977;123:60–62, with permission.)

the collateral ligaments to eliminate false inversion/eversion motion at that joint. The calcaneus is held in a cupped hand and moved in the axis of the subtalar joint, "down and in" and "up and out" (Figures 2-7, 2-8, and 3-9).

The other hand is used to note the motions at the midfoot and forefoot. It should not be used to attempt to move the subtalar joint, because hypermobility of Chopart joints (talonavicular and calcaneocuboid) can give a false impression of subtalar joint motion when none exists (Figure 3-10).

In my experience, this hypermobility of Chopart joints often develops in feet with solid talocalcaneal tarsal coalitions. It gives a false impression that a rigid flatfoot is flexible, not only when subtalar joint motion is incorrectly assessed manually, but also when it is assessed with toe standing (Figure 3-11).

The best way to improve your skills for assessing subtalar joint motion is to practice in the OR during a foot deformity correction operation while observing your technique and the resultant motions of the subtalar joint under mini-fluoroscopy.

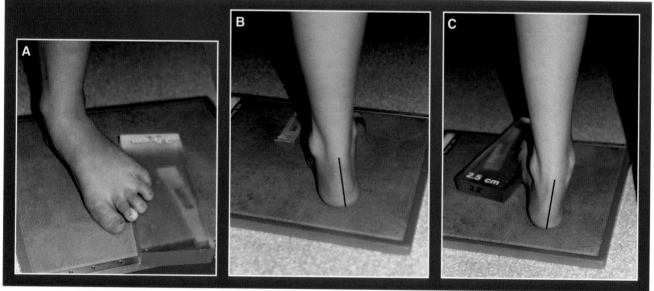

Figure 3-4. Modified Coleman block test. **A.** A 2.5-cm block of Plexiglas (or wood) is placed under the lateral 2–3 MT heads while keeping the heel on the ground. **B.** The posterior view with no block. The hindfoot is in varus. **C.** With the block under the lateral 2–3 MT heads, the hindfoot varus has converted to valgus, indicating flexibility of the subtalar joint. This can be confirmed radiographically (**see Assessment Principle #19, this chapter**).

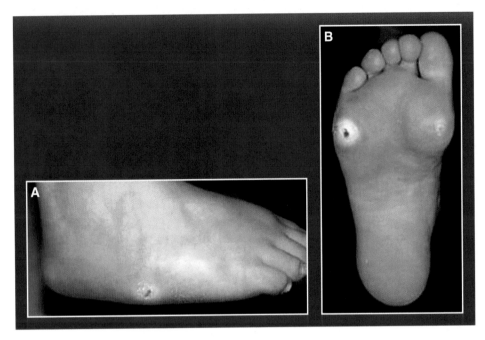

Figure 3-5. Exaggerated and unsafe skin pressures in the cavovarus feet of children with myelomeningocele. **A.** A cavovarus foot with hemorrhagic callus following healing of a neurotrophic ulcer. **B.** Deep neurotrophic ulcer with large surrounding area of thick callus formation under the 5th MT head and a recently healed ulcer under the 1st MT head.

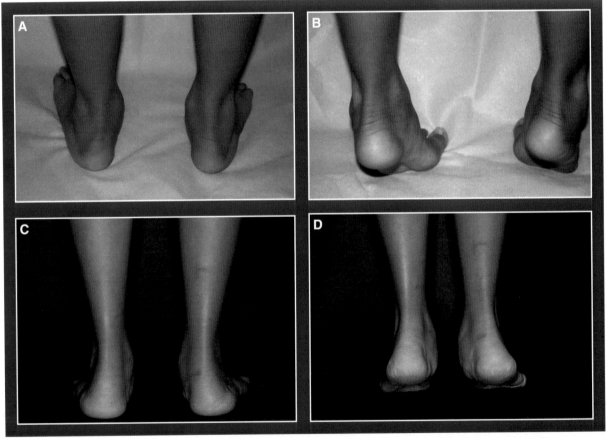

Figure 3-6. **A.** Flexible flatfeet with hindfoot valgus, forefoot supination, and the "too many toes" sign (toes seen lateral to the hindfoot when viewed from behind). **B.** With toe standing, the valgus hindfoot of a flexible flatfoot converts to varus, the arch elevates with reversal of the forefoot supination to pronation, and the toes appear medial to the hindfoot. **C.** Rigid flatfeet with the same segmental deformities as the flexible flatfoot, i.e., hindfoot valgus, forefoot supination, and the "too many toes" sign. **D.** With toe standing, nothing changes except that the heels elevate off the ground.

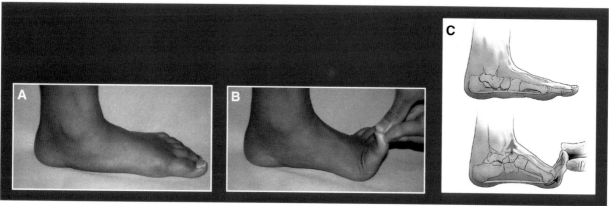

Figure 3-7. The Jack toe raise test, like toe standing, demonstrates hindfoot/subtalar joint flexibility in a flexible flatfoot **(A)** by means of the "windlass action" of the plantar fascia. The plantar fascia originates on the plantar aspect of the calcaneus and inserts into the plantar aspect of the toes through multiple interconnections. Great toe dorsiflexion **(B)** pulls the plantar fascia distally under the pulley of the head of the 1st MT. Since the plantar fascia is of fixed length, the great toe can only fully dorsiflex if the calcaneus is pulled distally toward the MT heads, thereby shortening the foot, elevating the longitudinal arch, and inverting the subtalar joint **(C)**.

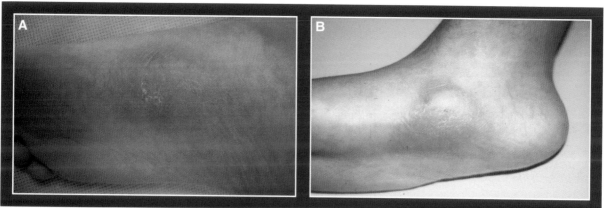

Figure 3-8. Contracture of the gastrocnemius or the entire triceps surae prevents the talus from dorsiflexing in the ankle joint. The calcaneus can dorsiflex past the plantar flexed talus by taking advantage of subtalar joint eversion—*dorsiflexion*, external rotation, and pronation of the calcaneus/acetabulum pedis. The talus remains rigidly plantar flexed while the navicular and the rest of the acetabulum pedis move "up and out," thereby concentrating all the weight-bearing stresses under the talar head **(A & B)**. Since the plantar flexion of the talus is unyielding, firm or rigid arch supports will increase skin pressure and pain at that site.

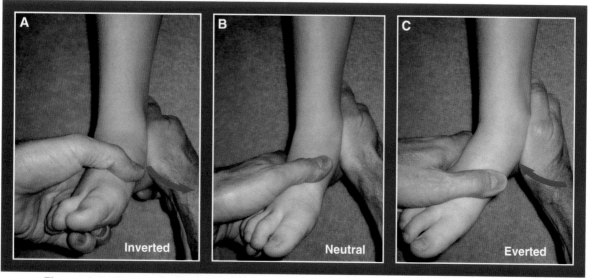

Figure 3-9. Attempt to move the subtalar joint "down and in" and "up and out" with a cupped hand on the heel, while maintaining the ankle at neutral dorsiflexion. Do not attempt to move the hindfoot with the hand on the forefoot because there can be excessive motion through Chopart's joints (talonavicular and calcaneocuboid) that gives the false impression of subtalar motion. Only use the hand on the forefoot to stabilize the foot and to detect false motions. **A.** Inverted. **B.** Neutral. **C.** Everted.

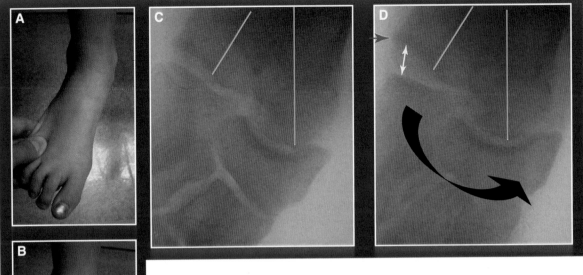

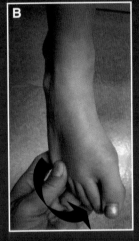

Figure 3-10. **A, B.** Foot with a large, solid talocalcaneal tarsal coalition and no motion possible between the talus and calcaneus, but apparent subtalar motion when examined incorrectly. The purple arrow points to a bony prominence that is noted with the forefoot "inverted" (actually adducted), but not apparent with the foot in its normal everted position. **C.** AP x-ray of the foot in its normal everted position. The dark blue lines are the axes of the talus and the calcaneus. **D.** The curved arrow shows the direction that the forefoot/midfoot was moved. The navicular has rotated into better axial alignment with the talus suggesting inversion of the subtalar joint, but there is no change in the relationship between the talus and calcaneus (see *dark blue lines*). Instead, the apparent inversion took place because of acquired hypermobility at the calcaneocuboid joint. Normally a nonmobile joint, the calcaneocuboid joint opened up like a book (*yellow double-headed arrow*). The bony prominence (at the tip of the *purple arrow*) is the anterior end of the calcaneus that has been exposed because of the plantar–medial movement of the cuboid, along with the navicular, at Chopart joints.

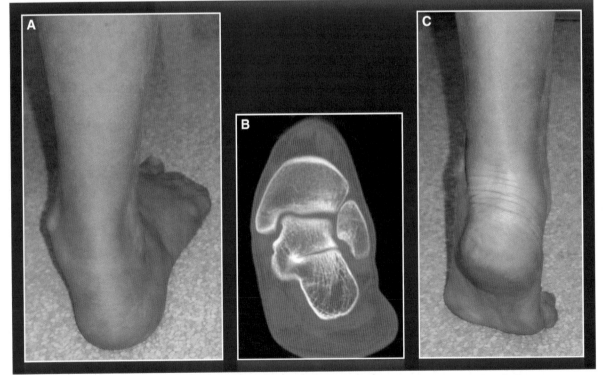

Figure 3-11. The same foot as in Figure 3-10. **A.** Valgus hindfoot with the "too many toes" sign. **B.** Coronal CT scan cut shows large osseous middle facet coalition, narrow posterior facet, and excessive valgus deformity. **C.** With toe standing, the hindfoot valgus deformity "corrects" to apparent varus, the arch elevates, and there are less toes seen laterally. This is a physiologic adaptation that can only happen because of acquired hypermobility at Chopart joints, specifically at the calcaneocuboid joint. The reason for the clinical appearance of hindfoot varus when the calcaneus is in rigid valgus alignment under the talus is unknown.

ASSESSMENT PRINCIPLE #11

An ankle joint deformity may coexist with a foot deformity, or it may be an isolated deformity. It must be differentiated.

The ankle joint is in valgus orientation to the anatomic axis of the tibia in all normal newborns. In otherwise normal children, the distal fibula and lateral distal tibia grow relatively faster than the medial distal tibia until about age 3 to 4 years. At that point, the ankle joint/tibial plafond becomes perpendicular to the tibia. It maintains that anatomic alignment through skeletal maturity (Figure 3-12).

That spontaneous change from physiologic neonatal ankle valgus to neutral alignment does not occur in children with myelomeningocele, lipomeningocele, early-onset poliomyelitis, other early-onset flaccid paralytic conditions, and approximately 66% of limbs with a clubfoot. The clinical assessment of ankle joint alignment and the differentiation from subtalar joint alignment are helpful in older children, particularly in those with the stated underlying conditions. In spastic conditions, such as cerebral palsy, normal spontaneous correction of neonatal ankle valgus to neutral occurs.

The lateral malleolus is longer/taller than the medial malleolus at all ages and in all underlying conditions (except fibular hemimelia). Therefore, with a valgus ankle joint, the distal tip of the lateral malleolus and that of the medial malleolus are in a transverse plane that is often perpendicular to the tibia (Figure 3-12A). When the ankle joint has assumed its adult alignment perpendicular to the tibia, the distal tip of the lateral malleolus is closer to the floor and further from the knee than the medial malleolus (Figure 3-12B). This assessment of the relative heights of the malleoli is helpful in the clinical determination of ankle alignment. It is particularly helpful in the clinical determination of the site of hindfoot valgus deformity, which can exist in the ankle joint, the subtalar joint, or in both joints. There may also be pathologic valgus in the ankle and varus in the subtalar joint, varus in both joints, or varus in the ankle and valgus in the subtalar joint. Radiographs of the ankle joint will confirm the specific anatomy (**see Assessment Principle #21, Figure 3-27, this chapter**).

The ankle joint can also have a procurvatum or recurvatum deformity. These are almost always acquired deformities. A flat-top deformity of the talus can occur following both nonoperative and operative treatment of clubfoot deformity, and results in a true or "functional" procurvatum deformity of the ankle (**see Anterior ankle impingement, Figure 5-1, Chapter 5**). Iatrogenic posterior distal tibial physeal arrest following clubfoot surgery can cause a true procurvatum deformity (**see Anterior ankle impingement, Figure 5-3, Chapter 5**).

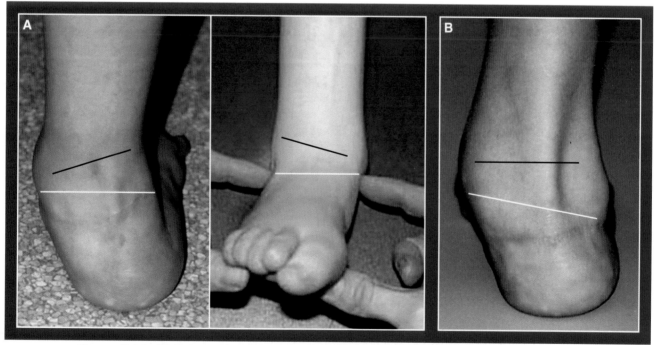

Figure 3-12. Clinical assessment of the relative heights of the lateral and medial malleoli relative to the floor can provide a clue as to the alignment of the ankle joint (varus or valgus). Yellow line connects the distal tips of the lateral and medial malleoli. Black line represents the plane of the ankle joint. **A.** The ankle joint is in valgus alignment relative to the tibia from birth until age 3 to 4 years, resulting in malleoli that are at the same transverse level. Those neonatal relationships persist in many paralytic conditions and a large percentage of clubfeet. **B.** The ankle joint is perpendicular to the tibia after the age of 3 to 4 years. The lateral malleolus is further from the knee and closer to the ground than the medial malleolus thereafter.

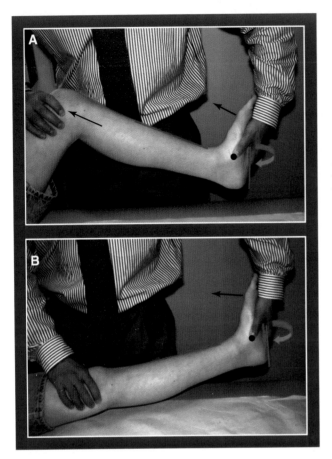

Figure 3-13. The Silfverskiold test. **A.** Testing the soleus and, effectively, the entire triceps surae/tendo-Achilles: 1. Flex the knee to relax the gastrocnemius (*black arrow* at knee). 2. Ensure that the talonavicular joint is in neutral alignment. If the subtalar joint is everted, as in a flatfoot, invert ("lock"—**see Basic Principle #7, Chapter 2**) the subtalar joint to neutral, and confirm anatomic subtalar joint alignment with a thumb over the plantar–medial aspect of the talonavicular joint (*black dot*). If the subtalar joint is inverted, as in a cavovarus foot, evert the subtalar joint to neutral. 3. Maximally dorsiflex the ankle joint (*black arrow* above foot) and record the angle between the plantar–lateral border of the foot (*red line*), which is the true proxy for the foot, and the anterior border of the tibial shaft (*red line*). *Do not* use the plantar–medial border of the foot as the reference line because supination or pronation deformity of the forefoot will give a false impression of ankle joint position. Ankle dorsiflexion greater than or equal to 10° is normal, as in this example. **B.** Testing the gastrocnemius: 1. While maintaining subtalar neutral, extend the knee to tighten the proximal end of the gastrocnemius. 2. The ankle will lose some dorsiflexion in most cases. 3. Record the angle between the plantar–lateral border of the foot and the anterior border of the tibial shaft. In this case, the ankle lacks about 5° of dorsiflexion from neutral, indicating contracture of the gastrocnemius.

ASSESSMENT PRINCIPLE #12

The presence of a gastrocnemius or an tendo-Achilles contracture must be identified and differentiated from each other.

Many foot deformities do not cause pain or functional disability unless they are accompanied by a contracture of the heel cord (the gastrocnemius alone or the entire triceps surae/tendo-Achilles). The ankle joint should have at least 10° of dorsiflexion with the knee extended and the subtalar joint in neutral alignment ("locked"—**see Basic Principle #7, Chapter 2**). The Silfverskiold test should be used to determine whether there is a contracture of the heel cord and, if so, whether the contracture is of the gastrocnemius alone or the tendo-Achilles. This will ensure that the proper tendon is lengthened if surgery is indicated, thereby avoiding under or overlengthening. The Silfverskiold test must be mastered (Figure 3-13).

The flatfoot presents a special challenge when determining contracture of the heel cord. The reason is that both the ankle joint and the subtalar joint dorsiflex and plantar flex (**see Basic Principles #6 and 7, Chapter 2**). The goal is to assess dorsiflexion at the ankle joint, i.e., the upward movement of the talus relative to the tibia. To do so, the subtalar joint must be anatomically aligned, or locked (**see Basic Principle #7, Chapter 2**), and stabilized by means of inversion to prevent subtalar dorsiflexion from being attributed to the ankle joint (Figure 3-13).

The cavus foot presents a different challenge to the assessment of a possible heel cord contracture. Cavus means plantar flexion of the forefoot on the hindfoot, i.e., equinus of the forefoot. Therefore, assessment of ankle equinus can only be performed by isolating the hindfoot. The forefoot should be obscured from your vision with your hand so that only the hindfoot can be seen (Figure 3-14).

ASSESSMENT PRINCIPLE #13

A detailed evaluation of strength, sensation, reflexes, and vascularity is required.

This is particularly true for the cavovarus foot, but is important for all foot deformities. Do not rely on EMG findings or on someone else to do it.

ASSESSMENT PRINCIPLE #14

The foot must be assessed clinically in weight-bearing, not just on the examination table.

Do this first to learn about the true deformities and functions/dysfunctions of the foot. The foot deformity will look very different when weight-bearing and non–weight-bearing. A flatfoot looks better than it truly is when it is not bearing weight (Figure 3-15).

And a cavovarus foot looks worse than it truly is when non–weight-bearing. Pain and/or disability are usually, if not

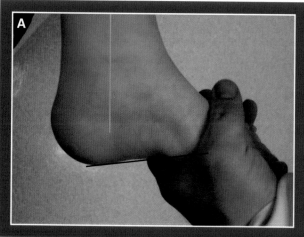
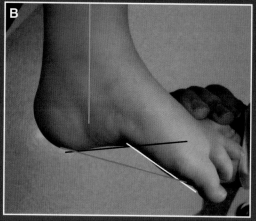

Figure 3-14. Assessing hindfoot dorsiflexion in a cavovarus foot. **A.** Evert the hindfoot to neutral (if possible), dorsiflex the foot, and extend the knee. Obscure the forefoot from your vision and assess hindfoot dorsiflexion. The vertical green line represents the axis of the tibia. The black line represents the inclination of the hindfoot. There appears to be ankle dorsiflexion above neutral, though it is somewhat limited in degree. **B.** With the forefoot exposed, the plantar aspect of the foot is represented by the red line. Using this line, there is an apparent significant lack of dorsiflexion of the foot at the ankle. In fact, there is lack of dorsiflexion of the forefoot (*yellow line*) in relation to the hindfoot (*black line*), i.e., cavus. One's eye is drawn to the position of the MT heads relative to the tibia which falsely gives the impression of equinus of the entire foot at the ankle. This foot needs correction of the cavus deformity alone. Inappropriate lengthening of the tendo-Achilles would convert cavovarus to calcaneocavus (**see Management Principle #23, Figure 4-19, Chapter 4**).

always, experienced when weight-bearing. Observation of the weight-bearing foot helps understand the pattern of pain and disability.

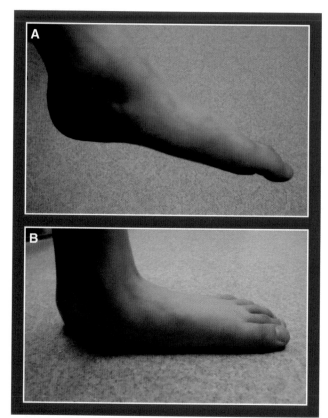

Figure 3-15. **A.** A severe flexible flatfoot seen dangling in space, with the child seated on the exam table with the leg hanging down. **B.** The same foot in full weight-bearing.

ASSESSMENT PRINCIPLE #15

If pain is a complaint, the child should be asked to point to the exact location(s).

By having the child identify the point(s) of maximal tenderness, you can start your physical examination away from that site(s) and learn about the surrounding area(s) before creating pain that might limit the rest of the examination. You can also quickly determine if your working diagnosis (based on the history) is valid even before you touch the foot (Figure 3-16).

ASSESSMENT PRINCIPLE #16

Signs and symptoms must match the presumed pathology, so ensure that you have enough information before focusing on a radiographic finding.

There are many common anatomic foot variations, such as tarsal coalitions and accessory naviculars, that do not cause

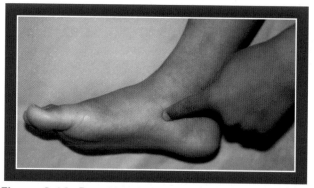

Figure 3-16. Exact identification by the child of the site(s) of pain is important.

pain or functional disability in the majority of affected individuals. Therefore, it is important to ensure that the signs and symptoms match those associated with the radiographic finding. If they do not, the two are unrelated and a more thorough investigation is required.

RADIOGRAPHS AND OTHER IMAGING

ASSESSMENT PRINCIPLE #17

All radiographs for the assessment of foot deformities should be btained in *weight-bearing,* or *simulated weight-bearing* if the former is not possible because of extreme youth or the child's inability to stand.

This is the radiographic version of **Assessment Principle #14**. The appropriate clinical assessment of foot deformities is performed in weight-bearing. Radiographs must, therefore, be obtained in weight-bearing to correlate the anatomic alignment of the bones and joints with the outward appearance of the foot. Recall that a flatfoot looks better than it truly is when it is not bearing weight (Figure 3-17).

And a cavovarus foot looks worse than it truly is when non–weight-bearing. Specialized views, such as oblique views, can be taken non–weight-bearing because they are used to identify anatomic abnormalities other than bone and joint alignment.

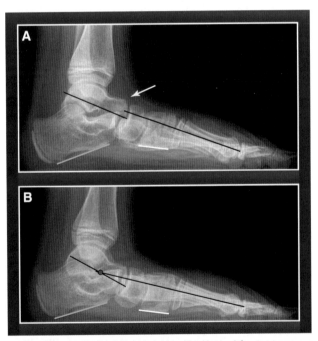

Figure 3-17. **A**. Partial weight-bearing lateral foot x-ray. Normal-appearing foot with straight talus–1st MT line. The white line indicates the plantar cortex of the medial cuneiform. The green line is the calcaneal pitch. The yellow arrow shows dorsal positioning of the head/neck of the talus in relation to the dorsal cortex of the navicular, a subtle sign of partial weight-bearing. **B**. Full weight-bearing lateral x-ray of the same foot. Note the plantar sag at the talonavicular joint with the foot-CORA in the talar head, the lowering of the calcaneal pitch, the plantar position of the plantar cortex of the medial cuneiform, and the level alignment of the dorsal cortices of the talus and navicular. These are all characteristics of a flatfoot.

The standard radiographic views for assessing foot deformities are *standing* AP, lateral, and (medial or standard) oblique; additional views include lateral oblique and Harris axial views.

ASSESSMENT PRINCIPLE #18

The foot-CORA (center of rotation of angulation) method should be used pre-, intra-, and postoperatively for the most objective evaluation of foot deformities and malformations.

For over a century, radiographs have been used to add objectivity to the clinical assessment of bones and joints and their alignment. The mechanical axis is the most basic radiographic measurement used to assess overall lower extremity alignment. A normal mechanical axis is one in which there is a straight line/linear relationship between the centers of the hip, knee and ankle. It is intuitive that, in a limb with a mechanical axis deviation (i.e., the centers of the three joints are not on the same line), one or more angular deformities exist at some point(s) between the hip and the ankle. It is perhaps less intuitive that, in a limb with a normal mechanical axis, two or more opposite direction angular deformities can exist. These intervening bone deformities can create joint malorientation, a feature of limb alignment that is as important to normalize as is the mechanical axis. Normalization of both features is important for the health and longevity of the joints.

Normative data exist for the shape of each of the long bones of the extremities. Those data were derived by quantifying the angle between the shaft of each bone and either the adjacent articular surface or the unique configuration of the end of that particular bone. An assumption is that the shafts of all long bones are straight, except for the femur in the sagittal plane.

Assessment of the site(s) of deformity within a bone is best done using Paley's CORA method. A line is drawn through the longitudinal axis of each straight segment of the shaft. These lines are related to each other as well as to the adjacent joint orientation lines. The site at which a normal and an abnormal, or an abnormal and an abnormal, segmental axis line intersect is a CORA. The CORA represents a static, fixed, structural deformity that exists within a bone. A CORA can exist in the epiphysis, the physis, the metaphysis, or the diaphysis. Using the CORA assessment principles, the site(s) of deformity can be determined and used as a guide for deformity correction. The CORA method can also be used to assess the success of deformity correction.

There are several justifications for a unique CORA method for assessment of foot deformities. The bones of the midfoot are (1) small; (2) irregularly shaped, without clearly definable axes; (3) hard to see/visualize and measure on radiographs, in part because they have overlapping shadows; (4) not ossified or not fully ossified in young children; (5) often not amenable to drawing axis lines because the ossification centers are spherical (note: the axis of a sphere is a dot, not a line); and (6) truly deformed in only a few conditions, including metatarsus adductus, metatarsus primus varus, skewfoot (only the forefoot deformity), and only the cavus component of cavovarus deformity.

Unlike the midfoot bones, the oval-shaped ossification centers of the hindfoot bones (talus and calcaneus) (1) are present at birth and (2) roughly represent the true shape of those bones, even in infancy, so that axis lines can be drawn fairly reliably. However, these two bones are more often malaligned than deformed.

Ossification of the MT bones represents the true shape of those bones, even in infancy. Axis lines can be drawn very reliably. Interestingly though, the MTs, like the hindfoot bones, are more often malaligned than deformed.

These features of the foot bones make it unreliable or impossible to apply the CORA method that is used for the long bones of the extremities to the assessment of foot deformities, particularly in children.

Normative, static radiographic measurements for adult foot alignment exist. They relate the axis of one long bone with another, such as the talus to the 1st MT, the talus to the calcaneus, and the calcaneus to the 4th MT. The talus is the stable structure around which the acetabulum pedis rotates on the fixed oblique axis of the subtalar joint (see Basic Principles #6 and 7, Chapter 2). The axis of the talus can be used as a linear proxy for the sagittal plane alignment of the ankle joint because the axis of the talus is perpendicular to the *axis* of dorsiflexion/plantar flexion of the ankle joint in the coronal plane. The 1st MT is the distal–medial extension of the calcaneus/acetabulum pedis block that rotates around the talus. The axis of the 1st MT can be determined with more accuracy and reliability than that of the calcaneus, so it can be used as a proxy for the calcaneus when relating the axis of the calcaneus/acetabulum pedis block to the axis of the talus. This is true unless there is a second deformity distal to the acetabulum pedis, as there is in a skewfoot (see below).

Deformities of the foot and ankle are typically due to exaggerated malalignments of the bones of the subtalar joint complex (varus/inversion and valgus/eversion) and the ankle joint (plantar flexion/equinus and dorsiflexion/calcaneus), rather than deformities within bones; however both may exist. Deformity correction in the foot and ankle most often involves realignment of the bones in the subtalar and ankle joints, rather than osteotomies of bones, though both may be necessary.

I have developed a modified CORA method, the "foot-CORA," to assess the sites of deformity in feet and ankles to more accurately characterize the deformities and to help ensure that they are corrected at those sites, if at all possible. The basis of the method is the assessment of the relationship between the axis of the talus and the axis of the 1st MT in the transverse (AP) and sagittal (lateral) planes and, to a lesser extent, the relationship between the axis of the talus and the axis of the tibia in the sagittal (lateral) plane.

The normal AP talus–1st MT angle ranges from 12° (abducted) to −10° (adducted), with an average value of 4° (abducted) (Figure 3-18).

I have observed that, on the standing AP radiograph of a foot with normal alignment, the axis of the talus and the axis of the 1st MT are either parallel and narrowly translated from each other or they intersect in the head/neck of the talus. In a foot with isolated valgus/eversion or varus/inversion malalignment of the hindfoot, the axes of those bones consistently intersect in the head of the talus or as far anterior as the talonavicular joint. The point of intersection of the axis

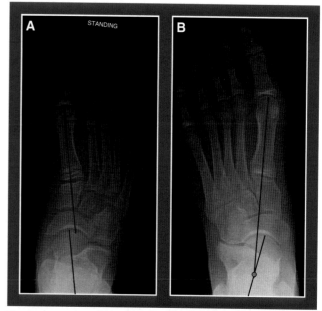

Figure 3-18. A. The axis of the talus and that of the 1st MT are parallel and narrowly translated from each other on this standing AP radiograph of a normal foot. B. The axis of the talus and that of the 1st MT intersect in the head/neck of the talus and are abducted less than 12° from each other on this standing AP radiograph of a normal foot.

lines can be considered a CORA. In contrast to a conventional CORA, this is a CORA *between* bones, rather than within a bone. In a foot with valgus/eversion deformity of the hindfoot, there is exaggerated abduction of the 1st MT axis in relation to the talar axis at the foot-CORA in the talar head (Figure 3-19).

In a foot with varus/inversion deformity of the hindfoot, there is exaggerated adduction of the 1st MT axis in relation to the talar axis at the foot-CORA in the talar head (Figure 3-20).

In contrast to the CORA in a long bone, an osteotomy is never performed at the subtalar foot-CORA. Instead, soft tissue procedures and/or osteotomies are preformed around the subtalar joint to align the axes of the talus and the 1st MT at the foot-CORA (Figures 3-19 and 3-20). The talus–1st MT angle can be used to quantify the degree of eversion and inversion deformity before and after correction.

It should also be acknowledged that there are some foot deformities in which the foot-CORA is within a bone. The two most common examples are metatarsus adductus and cavus, i.e. the forefoot plantar flexion deformity in a cavovarus foot. In both cases, the deformity is within the medial cuneiform (Figures 3-21 and 3-22).

The skewfoot, as well as some other unique deformities and malformations, presents a special challenge to the basic foot-CORA method that is resolved by the introduction of a new and unique axis line, the "tarsal line." It is a summary line, or proxy, for the overall alignment of the midfoot bones, which is otherwise difficult to assess due to the challenges noted above (the bones are small, irregular in shape, and delayed in ossification). Utilization of the tarsal line is particularly helpful when there are two opposite direction deformities between the talus and the 1st MT, as classically seen in

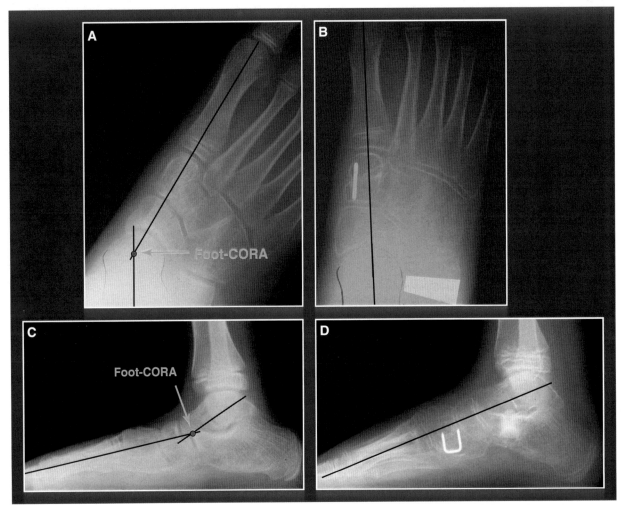

Figure 3-19. The foot-CORA for flatfoot. **A.** The foot-CORA for valgus/eversion deformity of the hindfoot is in the head of the talus on the AP x-ray. **B.** The eversion deformity has been corrected at the foot-CORA with a calcaneal lengthening osteotomy (*gray trapezoid-shaped graft* highlighted) (**see Calcaneal Lengthening Osteotomy, Chapter 8**). The axes of the talus and the 1st MT became aligned without actually doing anything to either of the named bones. The osteotomy was performed in a different bone, the calcaneus. **C.** The foot-CORA on the lateral x-ray is also in the head of the talus. **D.** The axes of the talus and the 1st MT became aligned in this plane as well following the calcaneal lengthening osteotomy. The allograft in the calcaneus appears to be healed, but not yet remodeled, in this early postoperative x-ray. Within a year after surgery, it was difficult to identify the graft on x-ray.

skewfoot deformities. The tarsal line is drawn from the point of intersection of the axis of the talus with the subchondral bone of the head of the talus to the point of intersection of the axis of the 1st MT with the subchondral bone at the base of the 1st MT. The tarsal line and the axis of the 1st MT are collinear when there is no deformity of the forefoot on the midfoot (adduction or abduction) in the frontal plane. The tarsal line and the axis of the talus are collinear when there is no deformity of the subtalar joint (i.e., no inversion or eversion) (Figure 3-23).

ASSESSMENT PRINCIPLE #19

Hindfoot flexibility in a cavovarus foot deformity should be assessed objectively with the radiographic equivalent of the modified Coleman block test.

The modified Coleman block test, and the justification for the modification, was described in **Assessment Principle #9, Figure 3-4, this chapter**. Objective assessment of the flexibility of the hindfoot in a cavovarus foot deformity can be documented with standing AP radiographs of the foot both off and on the block. The normal AP talus–1st MT angle ranges from 12° (abducted) to −10° (adducted) (**see Assessment Principle #18, Figure 3-18, this chapter**). Varus/inversion deformity of the hindfoot is characterized by exaggerated adduction of the talus–1st MT angle. Correction of the AP talus–1st MT angle to the normal range when standing on the block indicates flexibility of the subtalar joint (**see Assessment Principle #18, Figure 3-20, this chapter**), whereas incomplete correction indicates inflexibility (Figure 3-24).

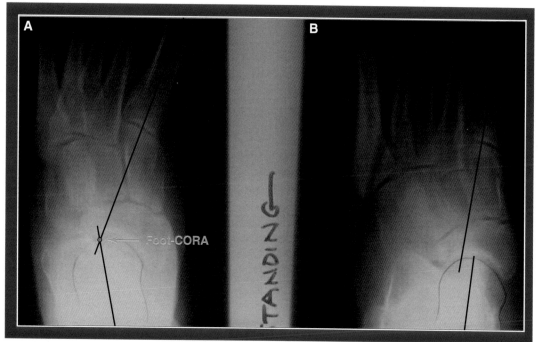

Figure 3-20. The foot-CORA for cavovarus. **A.** The foot-CORA for pure varus/inversion deformity of the hindfoot is in the head of the talus on the AP x-ray. In this example, there is mild associated metatarsus adductus which moves the foot-CORA slightly anteriorly to the talonavicular joint. **B.** The inversion deformity is flexible and has been corrected at the foot-CORA with the modified Coleman block test, as confirmed radiographically (**see Assessment Principle #19, this chapter**). The axes of the talus and the 1st MT became colinear without actually doing anything to either of the named bones. The same outcome follows plantar–medial soft tissue release of the subtalar joint (**see Superficial Plantar-Medial Release and Deep Plantar-Medial Release, Chapter 7**).

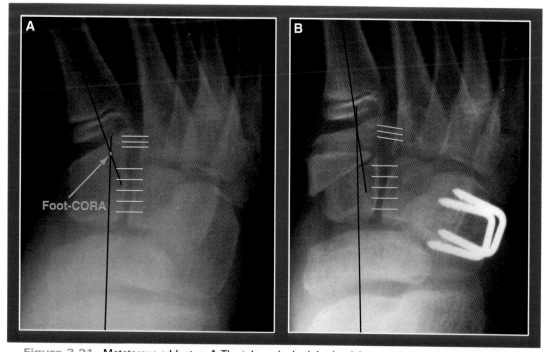

Figure 3-21. Metatarsus adductus. **A.** The talonavicular joint (and, by association, the subtalar joint) is well aligned. The axes of the talus and the 1st MT intersect in the medial cuneiform, indicating that to be the foot-CORA (*orange stripes* represent the interosseous ligaments). **B.** A medially-based opening wedge osteotomy of the medial cuneiform, along with a closing wedge osteotomy of the cuboid, has been performed. The foot-CORA has been improved significantly. The osteotomy began approximately half way from distal to proximal along the medial border of the medial cuneiform and angled slightly distal to end adjacent to the 2nd MT/middle cuneiform joint. Having created the osteotomy adjacent to that joint, the fragments have more mobility than if the osteotomy had ended more proximally adjacent to the medial cortex of the middle cuneiform. The interosseous ligaments maintained the appropriate amount of control of the fragments (**see Medial Cuneiform Osteotomies, Chapter 8**).

31

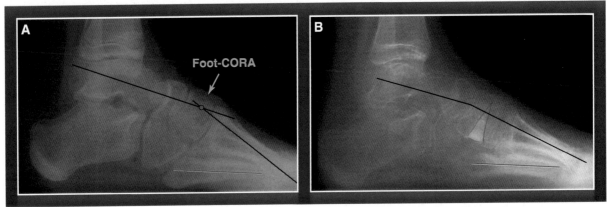

Figure 3-22. Cavovarus sagittal plane deformity. **A.** The foot-CORA on the lateral x-ray of a cavovarus foot is in the body of the medial cuneiform. This location indicates that the apex of the midfoot cavus deformity (not the hindfoot inversion/varus deformity) is within the medial cuneiform. Also note the exaggerated plantar flexion of the 1st MT in relation to the 5th MT (*purple line*). **B.** The axes of the talus and the 1st MT became aligned following a plantar-based opening wedge osteotomy in the medial cuneiform (**see Medial Cuneiform [Dorsiflexion] Plantar-based Opening Wedge Osteotomy, Chapter 8**). The angle between the 1st and 5th MTs became more parallel, the normal relationship.

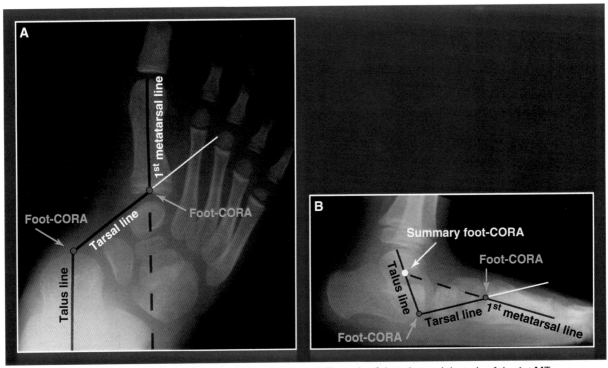

Figure 3-23. The foot-CORA method for skewfoot. **A.** The axis of the talus and the axis of the 1st MT are parallel, though severely translated, creating an angle between them of 0°. That would indicate no deformity, though significant deformities exist within this foot. The "tarsal line" helps to resolve this puzzle by creating a second foot-CORA. The talus–tarsal angle is abducted (+) at the posterior foot-CORA and the tarsal–1st MT angle is equivalently adducted (−) at the anterior foot-CORA in this foot. The opposite direction angles are added to each other when determining the summary talus–1st MT angle (0° in this example). The yellow line would represent the axis of the 1st MT if no midfoot/forefoot adduction deformity existed. In that situation, the talus–tarsal angle would be equivalent to the talus–1st MT angle. **B.** The axes of the talus and the 1st MT intersect in the body of the talus (*yellow dot*) far from the talar head, which is the foot-CORA in a pure flatfoot deformity. This is the summary foot-CORA and is indicative of a second deformity (second foot-CORA) between the talus and the 1st MT. The talus–tarsal angle represents the true subtalar deformity, which is much more exaggerated than the talus–1st MT angle suggests. The yellow line would represent the axis of the 1st MT if no midfoot/forefoot plantar flexion/cavus deformity existed. In that situation, the talus–tarsal angle would be equivalent to the talus–1st MT angle.

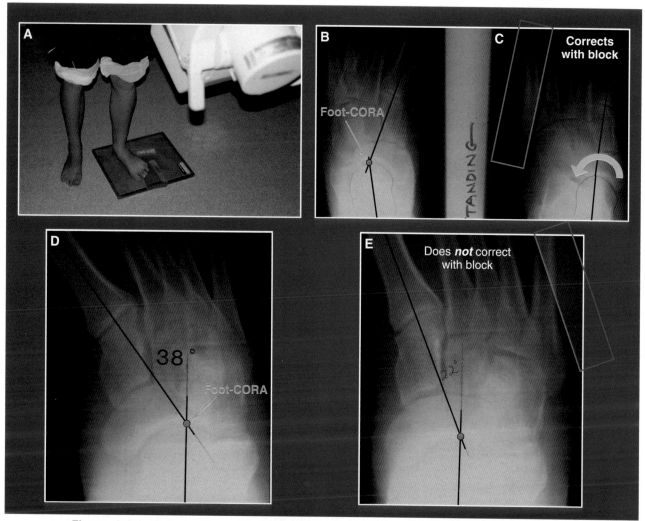

Figure 3-24. Radiographic modified Coleman block test. **A.** The patient stands with the lateral (4th and 5th) MT heads on a 2.5-cm block for an AP x-ray. **B.** Standing AP x-ray off the block. The talus–1st MT angle is adducted with the foot-CORA in the talar head, indicating hindfoot varus/ inversion. **C.** Standing AP x-ray on the block (*purple rectangle*). The talus–1st MT angle corrects fully, indicating a flexible subtalar joint. **D.** Standing AP x-ray off the block. The talus–1st MT angle is adducted with the foot-CORA in the talar head, indicating hindfoot varus/inversion. **E.** Standing AP x-ray on the block (*purple rectangle*). The talus–1st MT angle corrects only partially, indicating inadequate flexibility of the subtalar joint.

ASSESSMENT PRINCIPLE #20

There is usually a projectional artifact on the lateral radiograph of a foot with a varus/inverted or valgus/everted hindfoot deformity.

When a foot is C-shaped due to inversion or eversion of the hindfoot, the lateral x-ray beam cannot simultaneously pass perpendicular to the forefoot and the hindfoot. Therefore, order specifically positioned views to see each segment in a true lateral projection. The radiology technicians can easily visualize the forefoot and will generally aim the x-ray beam perpendicular to the MTs. That creates a rotational projectional artifact of the hindfoot in varus/inversion and valgus/eversion hindfoot deformities. Recall that one component of inversion is internal rotation of the subtalar joint/acetabulum pedis in relation to the talus/ankle which means, conversely, external rotation of the hindfoot in relation to the forefoot (Figure 3-25).

Also recall that one component of eversion is external rotation of the subtalar joint/acetabulum pedis in relation to the talus/ankle which means, conversely, internal rotation of the hindfoot in relation to the forefoot (Figure 3-26).

Finally, be aware that the best way to assess proper hindfoot positioning for a lateral radiograph is to note the relationship between the distal fibula and tibia. The posterior cortex of the distal fibula metaphysis and the posterior ossification margin of the distal tibial epiphysis are colinear in a true lateral x-ray of the hindfoot/ankle. It is unreliable to use the shape of the dome of the talus as a means to determine a true lateral projection because the ossification of the dome is not particularly dome-shaped in young children. Furthermore, there are many instances in which the dome had been crushed, devascularized, or otherwise injured, thereby, flattening its dome shape. And, as has just been discussed, flattening of the dome can be a projectional artifact. Therefore,

Projectional artifact–varus foot

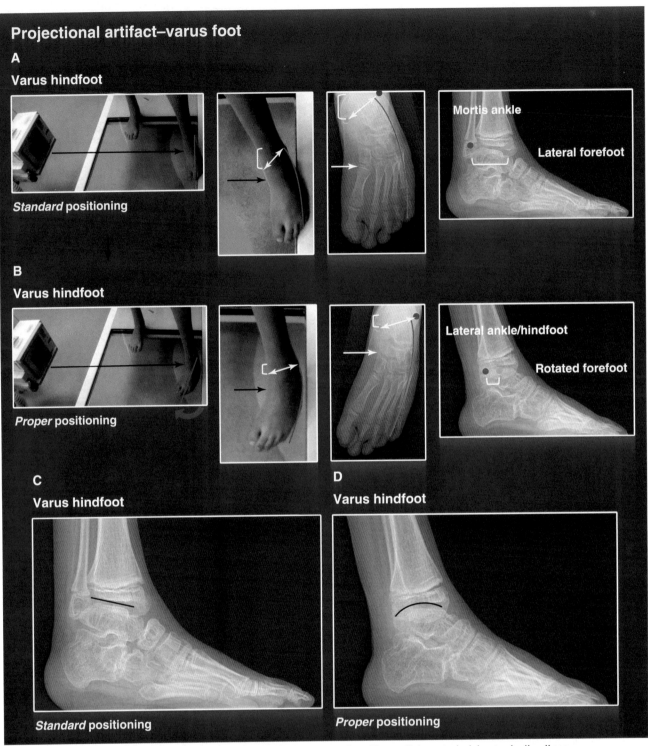

A

Varus hindfoot

Standard positioning

Mortis ankle

Lateral forefoot

B

Varus hindfoot

Proper positioning

Lateral ankle/hindfoot

Rotated forefoot

C

Varus hindfoot

Standard positioning

D

Varus hindfoot

Proper positioning

Figure 3-25. **A.** Standard positioning of a cavovarus foot: The radiology technician typically aligns the forefoot parallel with the plate (because the axis of the hindfoot is difficult to appreciate) and the beam perpendicular to the forefoot and plate. A true lateral image of the forefoot is obtained. Inversion of the subtalar joint includes internal rotation of the subtalar joint/acetabulum pedis in relation to the talus/ankle. That equates to external rotation of the ankle in relation to the forefoot—note positions of the malleoli (purple lateral malleolus and green medial malleolus)—and the radiographic appearance of an AP or mortis view of the ankle on the "lateral" x-ray of the foot. **B.** Proper positioning for assessment of the hindfoot: To see a true lateral image of the hindfoot/ankle, the technician must turn the forefoot toward the beam until the hindfoot is parallel with the plate (*purple curved arrow*). The forefoot image will look odd, but the hindfoot will appear as it should, with the posterior cortex of the distal fibula metaphysis in line with the posterior ossification margin of the distal tibial epiphysis. **C.** False appearance of a flat-top talus is seen in the standard positioning view. It is actually the normal talar dome appearance of a mortis view. **D.** The true talar dome appearance is seen when the foot is positioned properly.

Projectional artifact–valgus foot

A

Valgus hindfoot

Standard positioning

Rotated ankle

Lateral forefoot

B

Valgus hindfoot

Proper positioning

Lateral ankle/hindfoot

Rotated forefoot

C

Valgus hindfoot

Standard positioning

D

Valgus hindfoot

Proper positioning

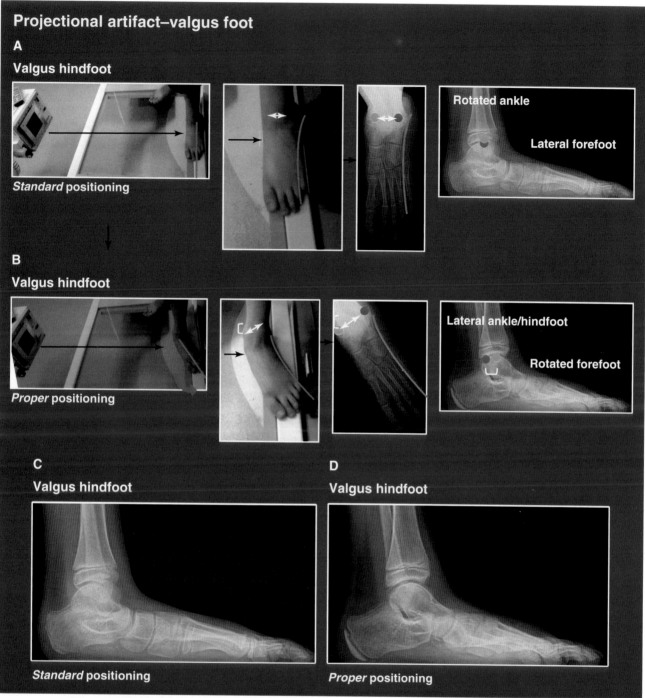

Figure 3-26. A. Standard positioning of a flatfoot: The radiology technician typically aligns the forefoot parallel with the plate (because the axis of the hindfoot is difficult to appreciate) and the beam perpendicular to the forefoot and plate. A true lateral image of the forefoot is obtained. Eversion of the subtalar joint includes external rotation of the subtalar joint/acetabulum pedis in relation to the talus/ankle. That equates to internal rotation of the ankle in relation to the forefoot—note positions of the malleoli (*purple* lateral malleolus and *green* medial malleolus). The lateral malleolus projects half way between the anterior and posterior cortices of the tibia. **B.** Proper positioning for assessment of the hindfoot: To see a true lateral image of the hindfoot/ankle, the technician must turn the forefoot away from the beam (*purple curved arrow*) until the hindfoot is parallel with the plate. The forefoot image will look odd, but the hindfoot will appear as it should, with the posterior cortex of the distal fibula metaphysis in line with the posterior ossification margin of the distal tibial epiphysis. **C.** Odd-shaped talus is seen in the standard positioning view. **D.** The true talus and talar dome appearances are seen when the foot is positioned properly.

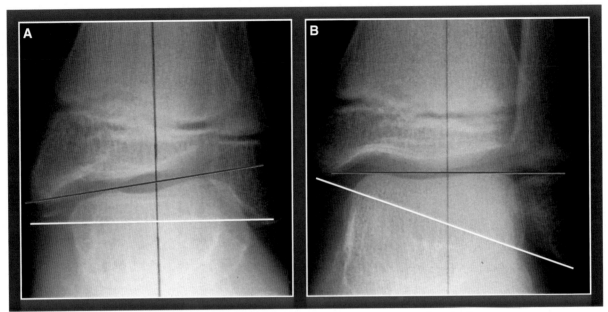

Figure 3-27. **A.** The ankle joint (*blue line*) is in valgus alignment at birth and gradually corrects to neutral; except it persists in many limbs with clubfoot and in those affected by paralytic conditions such as myelomeningocele, lipomeningocele, and poliomyelitis. The yellow line represents the distal tips of the medial and lateral malleoli, which are at approximately the same transverse level when the ankle joint is in valgus alignment. **B.** The ankle joint gradually becomes perpendicular to the tibia (*blue line*) and the lateral malleolus grows distal to the medial malleolus (*yellow line*) by age 3 to 4 years in normal limbs.

use the distal fibula to tibia relationships to determine if the projection is a true lateral of the hindfoot/ankle.

ASSESSMENT PRINCIPLE #21

Do not forget about ankle radiographs.

Ankle radiographs (standing AP, lateral, mortis) are not a standard part of every assessment of a foot deformity or malformation, but should be ordered if clinically indicated. The ankle joint is in valgus alignment at birth (**see Assessment Principle #11, this chapter**). The distal fibula and lateral distal tibia grow relatively faster than the medial distal tibia until approximately age 3 to 4 years, at which point the ankle joint is perpendicular to the tibial shaft. Neonatal ankle valgus deformity persists in children with paralytic conditions (such as myelomeningocele, lipomeningocele, and poliomyelitis) and in many children with clubfeet for unknown reasons. The ankle joint undergoes its normal conversion to neutral alignment in children with cerebral palsy (Figure 3-27).

ASSESSMENT PRINCIPLE #22

A CT scan in all three orthogonal planes and with 3D reconstruction is the best imaging modality for more detailed assessment of complex foot deformities and malformations. It is the imaging modality of choice to assess tarsal coalitions.

For most deformities and malformations, plain radiographs provide sufficient information to corroborate the physical examination findings. CT scans show the shapes of bones and the alignment of joints in three dimensions, the exact information needed to assess the more complex deformities and malformations, particularly those that have been operated on previously. MRI scans are best at the assessment of soft tissue pathology, which is not the intent of structural assessment. The exorbitant cost of an MRI (even in comparison with a CT scan) makes it fiscally irresponsible to obtain this study without careful consideration of the indications and the information desired, considerations that apply to all imaging studies. CT scans use ionizing radiation, but at a distance far from the most radiation sensitive parts of the body.

Importantly, the CT scan is the *definitive imaging study* for the diagnosis and management of talocalcaneal tarsal coalitions because the generally accepted criteria for choosing the appropriate treatment modality are based on CT scan findings (**see Talocalcaneal Tarsal Coalition, TCTC, Figure 5-2, Chapter 5**) (Figure 3-28).

ASSESSMENT PRINCIPLE #23

An MRI is rarely helpful or indicated for assessment of foot deformities and malformations, except in special circumstances.

Radiographs and CT scans are useful in assessing bone and joint abnormalities, specifically deformities and malformations. MRI scans are useful in assessing soft tissue abnormalities, but not as useful in assessing deformities and malformations. The exorbitant cost of an MRI of the foot might be justified in the assessment of a complex deformity or malformation in a very young child who has minimal ossification of the tarsal bones (Figure 3-29).

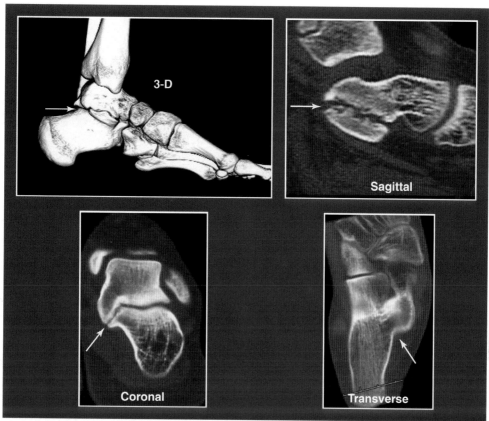

Figure 3-28. Collage of CT scan images of a foot with a middle facet talocalcaneal tarsal coalition (*yellow arrow*). The formerly healthy joint is narrow, sclerotic, irregular, and down-sloping.

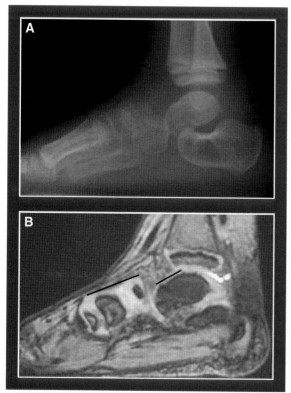

Figure 3-29. **A.** Lateral x-ray of a surgically treated clubfoot in a 3-year-old with a taller than expected midfoot and suspicion for dorsal subluxation/overcorrection at the talonavicular joint. **B.** MRI confirms dorsal subluxation/overcorrection at the talonavicular joint.

MRIs are the study of choice for soft tissue tumors and infections (Figure 3-30).

ASSESSMENT PRINCIPLE #24

A bone scan is a good and relatively inexpensive way to identify a specific site(s) of inflammation/pain, and is excellent at diagnosing complex regional pain syndrome.

There are many anatomic variations of the foot that, in many/most cases, do not cause pain. These include tarsal

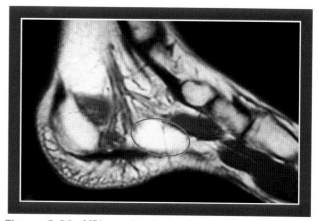

Figure 3-30. MRI reveals a lipoma (*purple oval*) in the tarsal tunnel in the abductor hallucis muscle that was compressing the medial plantar tibial nerve, creating pain and numbness in the distribution of the nerve.

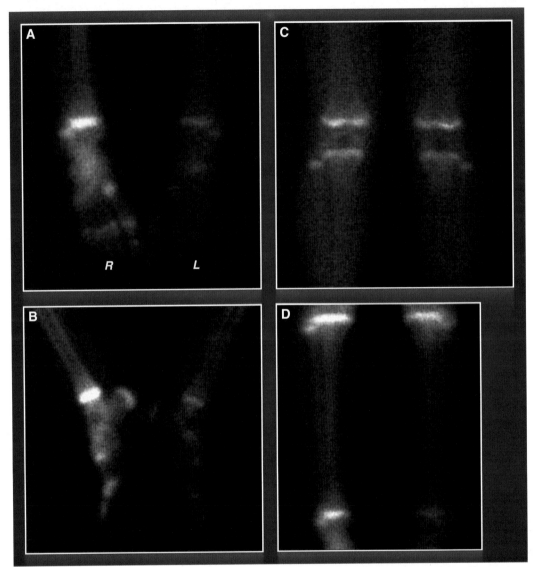

Figure 3-31. Bone scan demonstrating complex regional pain syndrome, a.k.a. reflex sympathetic or neurovascular dystrophy, pain amplification syndrome. **A.** AP image of the feet shows stocking–glove distribution decreased tracer uptake in the entire left foot and ankle. To the casual observer, and without benefit of the clinical history or visualization of the more proximal parts of the limbs, one might diagnose right foot and ankle pathology with generalized increased uptake. **B.** Lateral image of the feet confirms stocking–glove distribution decreased tracer uptake in the entire left foot and ankle. **C.** AP image of the knees shows essentially symmetric tracer uptake in the growth plates of the two limbs. **D.** AP image shows right-to-left symmetry of the proximal tibias/fibulas, but marked asymmetry at the ankles/feet with decreased tracer uptake on the left side.

coalition, accessory navicular, os trigonum, and a host of rare accessory ossicles. It is imperative to ensure that a radiographically identified anatomic variation is the cause of the pain and not merely an incidental finding (**see Assessment Principles #6, 15, and 16, this chapter**). A bone scan can be used to confirm if the anatomic variation is the source of the pain when the signs and symptoms are not characteristic for the anatomic variation that has been identified on physical examination, plain radiographs, and/or CT scan.

The bone scan should be ordered with magnified views and SPECT images in multiple projections. Both lower extremities must be seen for comparison, especially if complex regional pain syndrome is being considered, in which case there is most often a stocking–glove distribution decrease in uptake in the affected foot and ankle (Figure 3-31).

It is true that there is a theoretic risk of excessive radiation exposure to the gonads until the technetium is expelled from the urinary bladder, especially in females. But bone scans should be used infrequently and only for the rare indications stated. The alternative is to use an MRI scan, with its exorbitant cost and lack of specificity, to find the true site(s) of pain. The significance of "bone edema," which is frequently identified on MRI scans, is unknown.

Management Principles

MANAGEMENT PRINCIPLE #1

The decision (to operate) is more important than the incision (i.e., the surgical technique).

And the decision to operate on a foot deformity or malformation is based on (1) the known natural history of the condition, (2) the symptomatic and/or functional responses to nonoperative treatment (where appropriate), and (3) the reported risks and complications of surgery. A "well executed" operation for the right indication is far better for the patient than the "most skillfully executed operation in the history of surgery" for the wrong indication. The best surgeon is not necessarily the most skillful, but the one who knows when to operate. Of course, it is nice to make the best decisions and be technically excellent. We all strive for that combination of knowledge and skills.

MANAGEMENT PRINCIPLE #2

A less-than-ideal surgical or nonsurgical outcome can be due to a poor technique, a poor technician, or both.

This principle assumes that the patient satisfies reasonable indications for the technique in question. A surgical or non-surgical (e.g., Ponseti) technique is developed and, hopefully, tested by the originator before it is presented to the medical community. There is perhaps no technique that is so simple or foolproof that mere knowledge of the concept allows another surgeon to perform the procedure as well as the originator. And for some/many techniques, attention to all of the fine details of the procedure is critical for success. Failure to perform the procedure as described by the originator might result in a good outcome, but a poor outcome cannot automatically be attributed to the technique. It can, perhaps, be considered a poor technique only if other surgeons skillfully follow the fine details of the procedure (as published and

without modifications) and fail to achieve outcomes comparable to those achieved by the originator. Before abandoning or modifying a procedure that has been shown by others to be effective, make sure to perform it as described by the originator. Personal observation of, or tutoring by, an expert might be required, depending on the complexity and uniqueness of the technique. Though it is possible that the technique, as described by the originator, can be successfully performed only by the originator, such procedures should be extremely rare.

Admittedly, detailed descriptions for many of the procedures that are commonly and uncommonly performed are not published or otherwise accessible. I have included my time-tested techniques for many soft tissue and bony foot procedures in Chapters 7 and 8 of this text. Some are original to me, but most are my interpretation of the originals that often have not been well described in the literature. Some of the articles describing the original techniques can also be found in the bibliography in Chapter 9.

MANAGEMENT PRINCIPLE #3

You cannot un-operate on anyone.

Foot deformities and malformations are never lethal. Nonoperative treatment might prolong the temporary pain and disability, but might eliminate both, thereby avoiding the reported risks and complications of surgery.

MANAGEMENT PRINCIPLE #4

The (surgical) treatment could be worse than the condition itself.

No operation is without potential risks and complications that are unacceptable if the natural history of the condition or the response to nonoperative treatment provides favorable outcomes with little to no long-term disability. Nonoperative treatment corrects a high percentage of many congenital deformities (clubfoot, congenital vertical talus, and metatarsus adductus) and/or resolves pain and functional disability in a high percentage of certain other conditions (tarsal coalition, juvenile hallux valgus, and accessory navicular). Natural history trumps all treatment modalities. Many anatomic variations correct spontaneously through normal growth and development (flexible flatfoot, metatarsus adductus, and position calcaneovalgus) or persist without resulting in pain or functional disability (flexible flatfoot, metatarsus adductus).

MANAGEMENT PRINCIPLE #5

Modalities that *correct deformities:* (1) natural history, (2) physical stretching, (3) serial casting, and (4) surgery.

The natural history of congenital metatarsus adductus and positional calcaneovalgus is spontaneous correction in almost all cases (**see Basic Principles #3 and 4, Chapter 2**). Though perhaps better classified as an anatomic variation rather than a deformity, physiologic flexible flatfoot changes to an arched foot in most cases through its natural history.

Physical stretching exercises will increase the rate of dorsiflexion deformity correction for positional calcaneovalgus and will correct ankle plantar flexion deformity in many mild cases of congenital and acquired tendo-Achilles contracture. The technique for heel cord stretching in children with flatfoot/short tendo-Achilles must be performed in a specific manner to ensure that the proper structure, the tendo-Achilles, is stretched and that the proper joint, the ankle joint, achieves the increase in dorsiflexion. The reason was explained in **Basic Principle #6 and illustrated in Figure 2-7 in Chapter 2**. Dorsiflexion of the acetabulum pedis/calcaneus in relation to the talus, as seen in flatfoot deformity, is a component of eversion of the subtalar joint. Unless the subtalar joint is inverted to neutral and "locked" (**see Basic Principle #7, Figure 2-9, Chapter 2**), dorsiflexion stress will likely increase dorsiflexion/eversion through the subtalar joint rather than dorsiflexion in the ankle joint (Figure 4-1).

Serial casting can fully correct most cases of rigid congenital metatarsus adductus. It can fully correct most cases of congenital clubfoot and congenital vertical talus with the addition of minor surgery (Achilles tenotomy). And serial casting can correct some of the cases of congenital and acquired heel cord contracture that do not fully correct with physical stretching exercises. Serial casting can, at a minimum, partially correct foot deformities in children who are at even fairly advanced ages, so as to decrease the extent of required surgery.

Surgery is the final common pathway for foot deformities that do not correct spontaneously or respond fully to nonoperative treatment. Surgery involves soft tissue releases and/or plications, osteotomies, and, rarely, arthrodeses. Tendon transfers do not correct structural deformities.

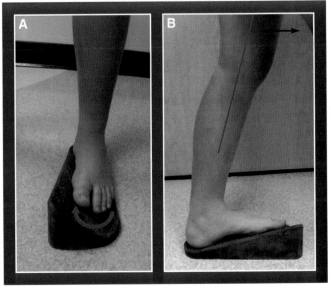

Figure 4-1. Heel cord stretching for a flexible flatfoot with a short tendo-Achilles must be performed with the subtalar joint inverted (**A**) and the knee extended (**B**). Recall that one component of eversion is *dorsiflexion* of the acetabulum pedis around the talus. If the subtalar joint is not inverted/"locked" (**see Basic Principle #7, Figure 2-9, Chapter 2**), it will merely further evert/dorsiflex, thereby stretching the medial soft tissues of the subtalar joint rather than the heel cord across the ankle joint. The knee must be extended to ensure that the gastrocnemius is also stretched at its proximal end as it crosses that joint. (Arch Safe™ Rubber biplanar wedge courtesy of Prasad Gourineni, MD with permission.)

As a corollary, natural history is the only modality that results in permanent deformity correction. There is a risk of deformity recurrence following all treatment modalities.

A commonly held belief by some health care professionals and most grandparents is that special "orthopedic shoes" and orthotics correct foot deformities in children. There is no scientific evidence to support that belief. The myth has been perpetuated because those devices have been credited with the deformity correction that has, in fact, occurred as a result of the natural history of the condition.

MANAGEMENT PRINCIPLE #6

Modalities that *correct dynamic deformities:* (1) focal injection of tone-reducing medication into muscles and (2) muscle-balancing tendon surgery.

Dynamic deformities are flexible; i.e., the joints can be passively moved through a full range of motion. They are due to muscle imbalance from underlying neuromuscular disorders in which there may be spasticity or weakness. Injection of botulinum toxin (BOTOX) into a spastic muscle has been shown to temporarily paralyze and weaken it, resulting in improved muscle balance across a joint. Although the effect is not permanent, it can be repeated. This is an appropriate treatment modality for a young child with spastic muscles in whom a delay in surgery until the child is older will often improve the results of muscle-balancing surgery.

Tendon lengthening/weakening and tendon transfer techniques are more permanent solutions to muscle imbalance, but they are not entirely reliable, predictable, or definitive. The main problem with a dynamic deformity is that it is the result of the problem (an underlying neuromuscular disorder) and not the primary problem (**see Basic Principle #12, Chapter 2**). After tendon surgery, the child still has the underlying nerve or muscle disorder. Therefore, recurrence of deformity and overcorrection are real possibilities (**see Management Principle #10, this chapter**).

MANAGEMENT PRINCIPLE #7

Modalities that *maintain deformity correction:* (1) focal injection of tone-reducing medication into muscles, (2) special shoes/braces, (3) orthotics, (4) physical stretching, and (5) balanced muscles.

Recurrence of a corrected deformity is common in many congenital and acquired deformities of the child's foot and ankle. In deformities caused by an underlying progressive neuromuscular disorder, recurrence is even more likely. Recurrence of a deformity is also common in children with underlying collagen disorders such as arthrogryposis and, at the other end of the spectrum, the ligament laxity syndromes. There are fewer recurrences in some deformities that are corrected later in childhood. However, delaying treatment is not always an acceptable option. The bottom line is that, unlike in adult foot surgery, maintenance of deformity correction in children and adolescents is a very important component of the overall treatment plan. It must be given consideration equal to the deformity correction itself and monitored long term.

Focal injection of tone-reducing medication into muscles can correct dynamic deformities and reduce the risk or rate of recurrence, but they do not guarantee maintenance of deformity correction because their effect is not permanent (**see Management Principle #6, this chapter**).

Special shoes/braces and orthotics do not correct deformities, but they are often helpful in maintaining deformity correction, even if worn only at night (Figure 4-2).

Daily stretching exercises are also an important modality for maintenance of deformity correction (Figure 4-3). The modified technique for heel cord stretching must be used for maintaining, as well as for achieving, correction in flexible flatfoot with short tendo-Achilles (Figure 4-1).

Surgically balanced muscles can maintain deformity correction, but achieving balance is an art and may not be achievable (**see Management Principle #22-4, this chapter**). Maintaining muscle balance is particularly challenging in progressive neuromuscular disorders (**see Management Principle #6, this chapter**).

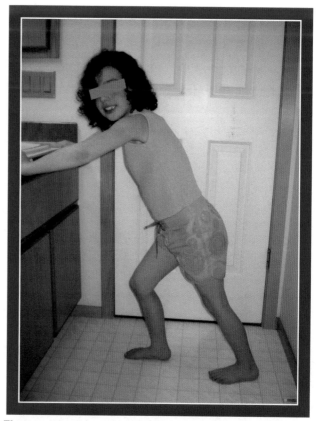

Figure 4-3. A few minutes of tendo-Achilles stretching can help maintain deformity correction after heel cord lengthening. A physical therapist is not required, except perhaps to teach the technique(s). Requesting that the stretching be performed immediately before or after brushing teeth (twice per day) could be the link that ensures compliance.

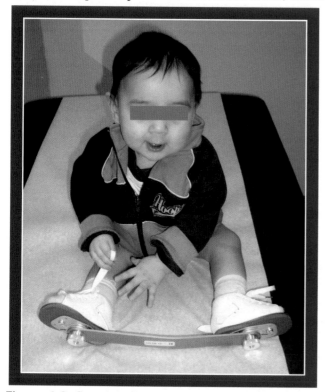

Figure 4-2. Foot-abduction brace worn at night for several years after clubfoot deformity correction using the Ponseti method.

MANAGEMENT PRINCIPLE #8

Treatment (nonoperative and/or operative) is indicated for:

1. *Congenital deformities and malformations that are known, or expected, to cause pain and/or functional disability unless corrected.*

These include congenital clubfoot, congenital vertical talus, rigid metatarsus adductus, rigid skewfoot, polydactyly, macrodactyly (Figure 4-4). They are treated well before they become symptomatic.

2. *Developmental and acquired deformities and malformations that are creating pain and/or functional disability.*

These include cavovarus foot, flexible flatfoot with short tendo-Achilles, idiopathic equinus, tarsal coalition, accessory navicular, spastic and paralytic foot deformities, iatrogenic deformities (Figure 4-5).

For both pain and functional disability, the treatment is disease-specific and can be nonoperative and/or operative.

MANAGEMENT PRINCIPLE #9

Surgical treatment is indicated for:

1. *Congenital deformities and malformations that do not, or cannot, correct with nonoperative treatment*

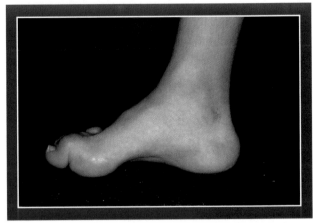

Figure 4-5. Cavovarus foot with claw toes in a boy with Charcot–Marie–Tooth disease. His feet were normally shaped, strong, and comfortable until 3 to 4 years prior to this photo. He presented with the obvious deformities along with instability, frequent ankle sprains, and weight-bearing pain under the 1st metatarsal head and the base of the 5th metatarsal on both feet. The natural history has been playing out for the last 3 to 4 years. There is no reason to believe that the pathologic changes will reverse or slow down. Therefore, there is no reason to delay treatment.

and are known to cause pain and/or functional disability unless corrected.

These include congenital clubfoot and vertical talus that do not respond to nonoperative (Ponseti and reverse Ponseti) management, macrodactyly, longitudinal epiphyseal bracket of the 1st metatarsal, polydactyly.

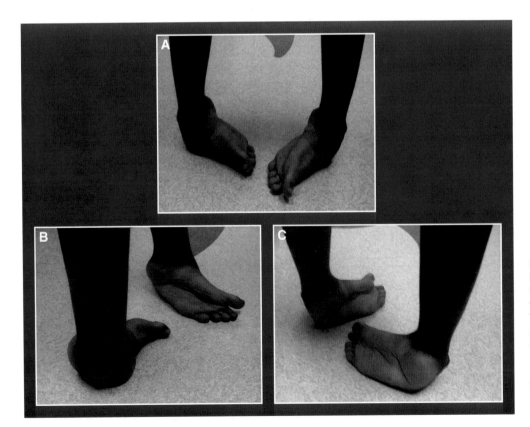

Figure 4-4. **A.** Front. **B.** Side. **C.** Back views of untreated congenital clubfeet in an 18-year-old male. They are unshoeable and are painful when walking on hard surfaces. Clubfoot never corrects without treatment. The natural history is well known. Early treatment can avoid disability in this common condition.

2. *Progressive cavovarus foot deformities that are associated with pain and/or functional disability.*

3. *Other developmental, persistent, and recurrent deformities that do not adequately respond to prolonged attempts at nonoperative treatment designed to correct the deformity, maintain deformity correction, relieve pain, and diminish or relieve functional disability.*

These include skewfoot, recurrent and overcorrected congenital clubfoot and vertical talus, idiopathic equinus, flexible flatfoot with short tendo-Achilles, tarsal coalition, accessory navicular, juvenile hallux valgus, spastic and paralytic foot deformities.

MANAGEMENT PRINCIPLE #10

Provide clear, accurate, and reasonable expectations to the patient and family of the short- and long-term outcomes of nonoperative and operative management.

Foot deformities and malformations are rarely "cured," i.e., made normal. But long-term comfort and function can be anticipated for many or most of them. Deformities attributable to neuromuscular disorders are the result of the problems and not the primary problems. Recurrence of deformity and the need for future treatment can be anticipated in many of these cases. Normal growth and development of a foot with a primary deformity can have an anticipated or unanticipated effect on the long-term outcome of the intervention. Share your predictions about future comfort and function and about the need for future treatment with the patient and family. That way there should be few surprises down the line.

MANAGEMENT PRINCIPLE #11

A surgical plan for each of the segmental deformities and muscle imbalances needs to be established before proceeding with surgery.

This means creating a list of the multiple related and unrelated procedures that are to be performed either during a single operative session or sequentially in cases of staged procedures. Some deformities are not evident until others are corrected. This needs to be anticipated before the start of the operation, based on one's knowledge and understanding of deformities, with a surgical plan ready for each additional deformity that might be identified intraoperatively. Be prepared, rather than surprised.

MANAGEMENT PRINCIPLE #12

Correct deformity at the site of the deformity. If that is not possible, use compensatory bone and soft tissue procedures.

That means:

1. Perform a calcaneal lengthening osteotomy (CLO) (**see Chapter 8**) rather than posterior calcaneal medial displacement osteotomy (**see Chapter 8**) for valgus/eversion deformity of the hindfoot. The former procedure (CLO) corrects all components of subtalar joint eversion at the site of deformity, whereas the latter procedure creates a compensatory deformity to correct valgus alignment of the hindfoot.

2. Perform a plantar–medial soft tissue release of the subtalar joint (**see Chapter 7**) rather than posterior calcaneal lateral displacement osteotomy (**see Chapter 8**) for varus/inversion deformity of the hindfoot. The former procedure corrects subtalar joint inversion at the site of deformity, whereas the latter procedure creates a compensatory deformity to correct varus alignment of the hindfoot.

3. Perform a medial cuneiform opening wedge osteotomy (**see Chapter 8**) rather than 1st metatarsal osteotomy (**see Chapter 8**) for cavus deformity (plantar flexion deformity of the 1st ray). The foot-CORA (center of rotation of angulation) for cavus (**see Assessment Principle #18, Chapter 3**) is in the medial cuneiform.

4. Perform a medial cuneiform opening wedge osteotomy (**see Chapter 8**) and cuboid closing wedge osteotomy (**see Chapter 8**) rather than metatarsal osteotomies or tarsometatarsal capsulotomies for metatarsus adductus. The foot-CORA for metatarsus adductus (**see Assessment Principle #18, Chapter 3**) is in the medial cuneiform.

When Willie Sutton was asked why he robbed banks, he said: "…because that's where the money is!" Go where the money is!

MANAGEMENT PRINCIPLE #13

Preserve joint motion (particularly subtalar joint motion) in the feet of children and adolescents by utilizing soft tissue releases/plications and osteotomies instead of arthrodeses.

Arthrodesis of the subtalar joint results in debilitating stress transfer to adjacent joints, particularly the ankle joint, leading to premature degenerative arthritis. Arthrodesis also has a detrimental effect on future growth and development of the foot. The subtalar joint is the shock absorber of the foot and, in fact, the entire lower extremity. Preserve its function at all costs (Figure 4-6).

MANAGEMENT PRINCIPLE #14

Use biologic, rather than technologic, interventions; i.e., rearrange and/or reshape anatomic parts rather than replace or interfere with them.

The overall reported short term complication rate of subtalar arthroereisis ("pseudoarthrodesis") with synthetic implants is 3.5% to 30%, with more recent reports of 3.5% to 11%. However, the actual rates are much higher if one includes the inappropriate implantation of these devices into normal physiologic flexible flatfeet, a practice employed by some

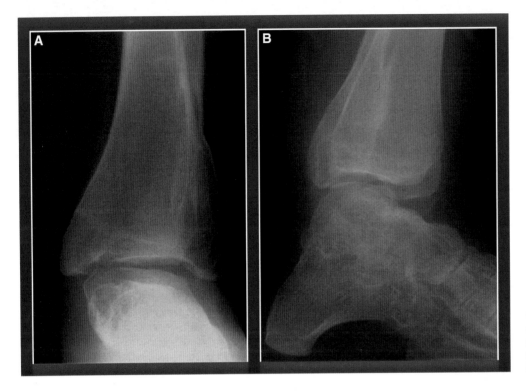

Figure 4-6. Degenerative arthrosis of the ankle joint several years after triple arthrodesis. **A.** AP x-ray. **B.** Lateral x-ray.

health care providers. Complications can be categorized as surgeon error, problems with biomaterials, biologic problems, and inappropriate implantations. Long term outcome studies have not been reported.

MANAGEMENT PRINCIPLE #15

Correct deformities *and* balance muscle forces.

1. *Deformity correction will not correct muscle imbalance.*

Deformity correction without muscle balancing can result in recurrent deformity. If muscle imbalance created the deformity, as is usually the case in cavovarus foot deformities, persistence of the muscle imbalance will recreate the deformity despite adequate initial deformity correction.

2. *Tendon transfers will not correct structural deformities.*

Muscle balancing without deformity correction will create a balanced deformity. That is not the goal (**see Management Principle #22-2, this Chapter**).

MANAGEMENT PRINCIPLE #16

Principles of cavovarus deformity correction:

1. *Release the plantar–medial soft tissues to realign the subtalar joint.*

The default position of the subtalar joint is valgus/everted (**see Basic Principle #9, Chapter 2**); release of the plantar–medial soft tissues (**see Chapter 7**) will result in partial or complete correction of varus/inversion. The subtalar joint is inverted in a cavovarus foot deformity, just as it is in a clubfoot. On the basis of the segmental deformities, one could consider an (equino-)cavovarus foot deformity an "acquired" clubfoot. One would never consider performing compensatory osteotomies or arthrodeses before attempting subtalar joint release and alignment in a clubfoot. The same approach should be used for a cavovarus deformity.

2. *Perform osteotomies to correct residual bone deformities.*

Depending on the severity and rigidity of the subtalar joint inversion deformity, plantar–medial soft tissue release might not be sufficient to realign the subtalar joint. In those cases, one or more hindfoot osteotomies (**see Chapter 8**) are required to correct the residual varus deformity. They should not, however, be used primarily in place of the plantar–medial soft tissue release.

Furthermore, alignment of the hindfoot does not correct the forefoot pronation deformity, which is a separate deformity that requires its own treatment (**see Basic Principle #5, Chapter 2**), specifically a dorsiflexion osteotomy of the medial cuneiform (**see Chapter 8**).

3. *Reserve arthrodesis of the subtalar joint as a salvage procedure.*

Most cavovarus deformities can be corrected with a combination of soft tissue releases and osteotomies. Arthrodesis of the subtalar joint can and should be avoided in children and adolescents (**see Management Principle #13, this chapter**) unless there is advanced arthritis in that joint, a rare finding in children and adolescents.

MANAGEMENT PRINCIPLE #17

Principles of planovalgus deformity correction:

1. *Perform osteotomies to correct bone deformities and/or align the subtalar joint.*

The default position of the subtalar joint is valgus/everted (**see Basic Principle #9, Chapter 2**). Therefore, release of the lateral soft tissues will result in no change in the eversion deformity, and plication of the plantar–medial soft tissues will not maintain deformity correction. The calcaneal lengthening osteotomy (**see Chapter 8**) corrects all components of valgus/eversion deformity of the subtalar joint at the site of deformity. The posterior calcaneus medial displacement osteotomy (**see Chapter 8**) corrects valgus alignment of the hindfoot *without* correcting the other components of eversion deformity. Specifically, it does not correct the dorsiflexion and external rotation malalignment at the talonavicular joint. The posterior calcaneus medial displacement osteotomy, when combined with other procedures, has a role in the correction of some specific planovalgus deformities.

Alignment of the hindfoot does not correct the forefoot supination deformity, which is a separate deformity that requires its own treatment (**see Basic Principle #5, Chapter 2**), specifically a plantar flexion osteotomy of the medial cuneiform (**see Chapter 8**).

2. *Plicate soft tissues to further stabilize the subtalar joint.*

Following correction of the eversion deformity of the subtalar joint with the CLO, the plantar–medial talonavicular joint capsule and the posterior tibialis tendon are lax. They should be tightened by means of a plantar–medial plication (**see Chapter 7**) to take up the redundancy in the capsule and to reset the muscle tension.

3. *Reserve arthrodesis of the subtalar joint as a salvage procedure.*

Most planovalgus deformities can be corrected with a combination of osteotomies and soft tissue plications. Arthrodesis of the subtalar joint can and should be avoided in children and adolescents (**see Management Principle #13, Chapter 4**) unless there is advanced arthritis in that joint, a rare finding in children and adolescents.

MANAGEMENT PRINCIPLE #18

The calcaneocuboid joint is the most distal site at which the lateral column of the foot can be shortened or lengthened to realign the talonavicular joint/acetabulum pedis in a foot with a varus/inverted or a valgus/everted hindfoot deformity. The body of the cuboid is too far distal.

The talonavicular and calcaneocuboid joints are collectively known as Chopart joints. The talonavicular joint is the anteromedial extent of the acetabulum pedis. As such, the navicular, along with the rest of the acetabulum pedis, rotates around the axis of the subtalar joint, i.e., "down and in" for inversion and "up and out" for eversion (**see Basic Principles #6 and 7, Chapter 2**). The calcaneocuboid joint, on the other hand, is a fairly nonmobile joint *within* the acetabulum pedis, analogous to the transverse limb of the triradiate cartilage *within* the acetabulum in the ilium (**see Basic Principle #7, Figure 2-11, Chapter 2**). The body of the cuboid, on the other hand, is distal to Chopart joints and the acetabulum pedis.

Plantar–medial soft tissue release of a varus/inverted hindfoot will produce partial-to-complete eversion of the subtalar joint with realignment of the talonavicular joint. In a long-standing deformity, full correction and realignment might not be possible because secondary bone deformity, manifest as a long lateral column of the foot, has developed. In such a case, there is residual inversion following a deep plantar-medial release (**see Chapter 7**). The long lateral column of the foot can be shortened to pull the navicular dorsolaterally to align with the talar head. Three procedures are effective in accomplishing this: the Evans calcaneocuboid joint resection/arthrodesis, the Lichtblau anterior calcaneus resection, and an anterior calcaneus lateral closing wedge osteotomy (**see Chapter 8 for a description of each procedure**). They are most commonly employed to treat resistant, residual, or recurrent hindfoot varus in clubfoot deformities in older children. A closing wedge osteotomy of the cuboid (**see Chapter 8**) is too far distal to affect the relationship between the navicular and the head of the talus. Its primary action is to help correct metatarsus adductus, particularly when combined with a medial opening wedge osteotomy of the medial cuneiform (**see Chapter 8**) (Figure 4-7).

In contrast to a foot with a varus/inverted hindfoot deformity, the lateral column of a foot with a valgus/everted hindfoot deformity is too short. The CLO (**see Chapter 8**) corrects valgus/eversion deformity of the hindfoot at the site of deformity and realigns the entire subtalar joint complex, including the talonavicular joint. An opening wedge osteotomy of the cuboid is too far anterior to affect bone relationships within the subtalar joint complex. Its primary action is to help correct metatarsus abductus (if, in fact, there exists such a deformity), particularly when combined with a medial closing wedge osteotomy of the medial cuneiform (Figure 4-8).

MANAGEMENT PRINCIPLE #19

When considering a dorsiflexion or plantar flexion osteotomy of the medial cuneiform for the correction of forefoot pronation or supination, one should also consider the alignment in the transverse plane (adduction or abduction).

The medial cuneiform has been recognized for some time as being the ideal site for correcting metatarsus adductus (**see Chapter 5**) with a medially-based opening wedge osteotomy, often combined with a closing wedge osteotomy of the cuboid. It is the foot-CORA for that deformity (**see Assessment**

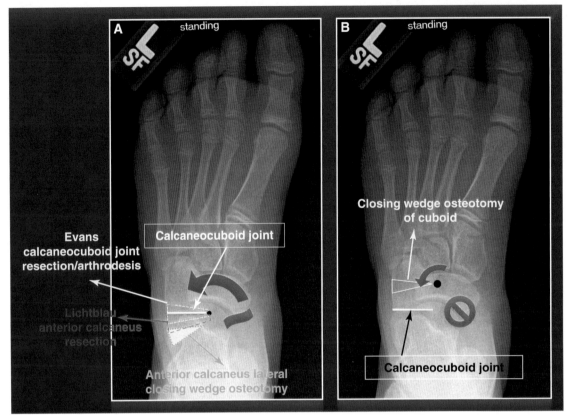

Figure 4-7. Lateral column shortening in a cavovarus foot. **A.** Following a deep plantar-medial release (*wavy red line*) (**see Chapter 7**), there may be residual inversion of the subtalar joint. The Evans calcaneocuboid resection/arthrodesis, the Lichtblau anterior calcaneus resection, and the anterior calcaneus lateral closing wedge osteotomy (**see Chapter 8 for a description of each procedure**) are all capable of shortening the lateral column of the foot and, thereby, correcting residual inversion of the subtalar joint with realignment of the navicular on the head of the talus (*curved purple arrow*). The black dot in the head of the talus represents the foot-CORA of the subtalar joint (**see Assessment Principle #18, Chapter 3**) around which the acetabulum pedis rotates following each of these three osteotomies. **B.** A closing wedge osteotomy of the cuboid (**see Chapter 8**) does not affect bone relationships in the subtalar or talonavicular joints (⊘). Its foot-CORA (*black dot*) is the medial cortex of the cuboid. In this foot, a closing wedge osteotomy of the cuboid would not realign the navicular on the head of the talus, but merely create a compensatory abduction deformity (*curved purple arrow*) distal to the true deformity in the subtalar joint (**see Management Principle #12, this chapter**).

Principle #18, Figure 3-21, Chapter 3). Less well recognized or acknowledged is the fact that the medial cuneiform is the foot-CORA for forefoot pronation (i.e. cavus) and supination (**see Assessment Principle #18, Figure 3-22, Chapter 3**). The base of the 1st MT is *not* the site of deformity (foot-CORA) for any forefoot or midfoot deformity.

Osteotomies in the medial cuneiform can, in fact, be used to correct forefoot pronation and supination, midfoot adduction and abduction, as well as combinations of those deformities (**see Medial Cuneiform Osteotomies, Chapter 8**). The medial cuneiform is, therefore, the workhorse of the medial column of the foot.

When treating pronation (plantar flexion of the 1st ray) and supination (dorsiflexion of the 1st ray) deformities of the forefoot, it is important to recognizing the alignment of the midfoot, i.e., adduction or abduction. Knowledge of this second plane alignment can help determine whether an opening or closing wedge osteotomy should be used to correct not

only the rotational deformity (pronation or supination), but also the angular deformity (adduction or abduction), or at least avoid exaggerating the deformity in that second plane.

The medial cuneiform is bordered laterally by two bones (the base of the second metatarsal and the middle cuneiform) and a joint (the second metatarsal–middle cuneiform joint) with interosseous ligaments along its entire border. The medial border is merely covered by soft tissues (skin, fat, and the anterior tibialis tendon). These features of the local anatomy of the medial cuneiform create four biplanar osteotomy scenarios (Figure 4-9).

1. A medial cuneiform dorsiflexion plantar-based opening wedge osteotomy (MC-DF-OWO) will always additionally create slight abduction, because the lateral ligaments create a tether on the two bone fragments that is not created medially. This would be best for forefoot pronation in cavovarus and skewfoot deformities. The base of the wedge is positioned plantar–medially in a skewfoot.

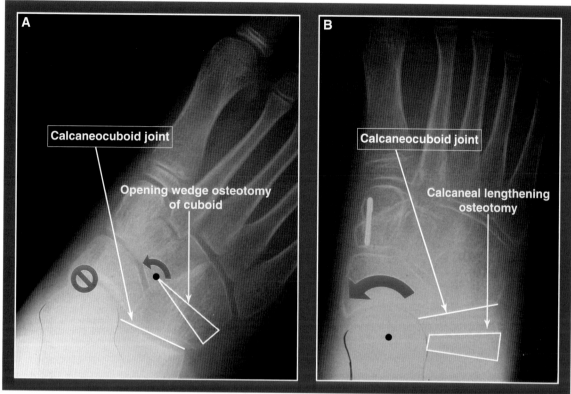

Figure 4-8. Lateral column lengthening in a flatfoot. **A.** An opening wedge osteotomy of the cuboid does not affect the relationship between the navicular and the talus (⊘) or correct eversion deformity of the subtalar joint. Its foot-CORA (*black dot*) is the medial cortex of the cuboid. It merely creates a compensatory adductus deformity (*curved purple arrow*) anterior to the true deformity in the subtalar joint. **B.** The calcaneal lengthening osteotomy (**see Chapter 8**) lengthens the lateral column of the foot and, thereby, corrects all components of eversion deformity of the subtalar joint with realignment of the navicular on the head of the talus. The black dot in the head of the talus represents the foot-CORA of the subtalar joint (**see Assessment Principle #18, Chapter 3**) around which the acetabulum pedis rotates following a CLO (*curved purple arrow*). This can also be accomplished by a distraction arthrodesis of the calcaneocuboid joint, which is unnecessary in children and adolescents, but preferred by some surgeons for the correction of the painful adult flatfoot.

2. A medial cuneiform plantar flexion plantar-based closing wedge osteotomy (MC-PF-CWO) will always additionally create slight adduction, because the lateral ligaments create a tether on the two bone fragments that is not created medially. This may be best for forefoot supination with no midfoot adduction deformity in flatfoot and dorsal bunion deformities.

3. A medial cuneiform plantar flexion dorsally-based opening wedge osteotomy (MC-PF-OWO) will always additionally create slight abduction, because the lateral ligaments create a tether on the two bone fragments that is not created medially. This would be best for forefoot supination with mild-to-severe midfoot adduction in flatfoot, skewfoot, and dorsal bunion deformities. It should not be used for typical flatfoot with neutral to slight abduction deformity of the midfoot. The additional abduction is undesirable.

4. A medial cuneiform dorsiflexion dorsally-based closing wedge osteotomy (MC-DF-CWO) will always additionally create slight adduction, because the lateral ligaments create a tether on the two bone fragments that is not created medially. This may be best for forefoot pronation (cavus)

with midfoot abduction, a combination rarely seen, except perhaps as an iatrogenic deformity. It should not be used for typical cavovarus with neutral to slight adduction deformity of the midfoot. The additional adduction is undesirable.

MANAGEMENT PRINCIPLE #20

Principles for distal tibia and fibula deformity correction osteotomies (see Distal Tibia and Fibula Varus, Valgus, Flexion, Extension, Rotational Osteotomies, Chapter 8):

1. *The fibula must be cut in conjunction with all distal tibial deformity correcting osteotomies. The reasons are based on geometry and the CORA principles* (Figures 4-10 and 4-11).

When correcting angular and/or rotational deformities of the tibia and fibula, the goal is to align the central axes of the proximal and distal tibial fragments, thereby centering the ankle directly under the knee. This means that the central

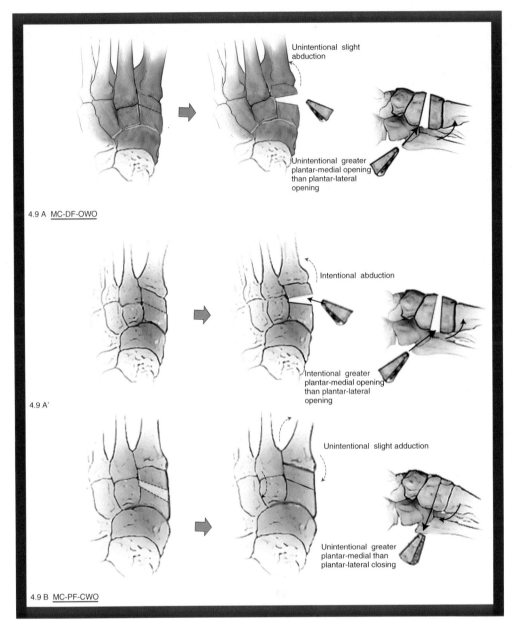

Figure 4-9. Medical cunieform dorsiflexion and plantar flexion osteotomies. Curved purple arrows on AP images show unintentional and intentional changes that occur in the frontal plane (adduction or abduction) when these osteotomies are performed **(see text)**. Curved black arrows on the lateral images show the intentional dorsiflexion and plantar flexion changes that occur. **A. Medial cuneiform (dorsi-flexion) plantar-based opening wedge osteotomy (MC-DF-OWO).** This is best for a *cavovarus* deformity, as it corrects forefoot pronation (plantar flexion of the 1st ray) and adds some unintentional, yet acceptable, midfoot abduction to the abduction/eversion that is being achieved in the hindfoot with the plantar-medial soft tissue release. This frontal plane deviation is due to the tethering effect of the bones and ligaments on the lateral side of the medial cunieform fragments, an effect that is observed with all medial cunieform osteotomies despite attempts to create pure sagittal plane correction. A'. Consideration of both planes and tha lateral tethering effects are also useful for a *skewfoot with* adduction/pronation deformities of the forefoot/midfoot. Intentional plantar-medial alignment of the base of the wedge will correct both deformities simultaneously. **B. Medial cuneiform (plantar flexion) plantar-based closing wedge osteotomy (MC-PF-CWO).** This is best for a *flatfoot,* as it corrects forefoot supination (dorsiflexion of the 1st ray) and adds some unintentional, yet acceptable, midfoot adduction to the adduction/inversion that is being achieved in the hindfoot with the calcaneal lengthening osteotomy. It is also useful for a *dorsal bunion with* no midfoot angular deformity.

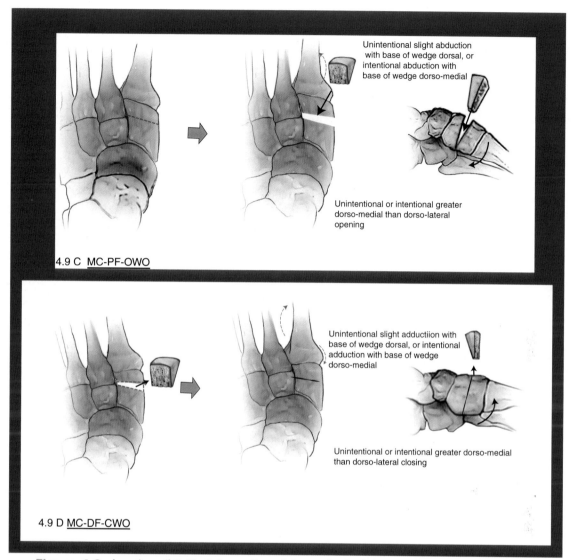

4.9 C MC-PF-OWO

4.9 D MC-DF-CWO

Figure 4-9. *(continued)* C. **Medial cuneiform (plantar flexion) dorsal-based opening wedge osteotomy (MC-PF-OWO).** This is best for: a *skewfoot with* adduction/supination deformities (align the base of the wedge dorsomedially); a *dorsal bunion with* midfoot adduction; and possibly a *flatfoot with* forefoot supination *and* mild midfoot *adduction* (if neutral or abducted, the additional abduction might be undesirable). D. **Medial cuneiform (dorsi-flexion) dorsal-based closing wedge osteotomy (MC-DF-CWO).** This is best for forefoot pronation (cavus) *and* midfoot abduction, a combination rarely seen, except perhaps as an iatrogenic deformity. If used for a typical cavus deformity with neutral or slight adduction deformity, the unintentional additional adduction might be undesirable.

axes of the proximal and distal fibula fragments can never be aligned. Therefore, without an osteotomy, the fibula will resist tibial deformity correction.

More specifically, for angular deformity correction, the tibial osteotomy is rarely performed at the CORA, which in children is usually the growth plate. Therefore, translation of the fragments is required and, geometrically, the fibula must translate even further than the tibia.

Furthermore, the lateral tibial cortex is never the apex or base of the angular deformity. It is the intended apex or base of the deformity *correction*. The lateral cortex of the fibula is the apex or base of the deformity. Without a fibula osteotomy, the tibial osteotomy surfaces will not meet.

2. *Consider the intended direction of movement of the distal tibial fragment to determine the proper plane for the fibula osteotomy* (**Figures 4-12 and 4-13**).

The fibula should be cut obliquely to create broad surfaces for rapid healing because, as discussed above, the ends will not be in exact or direct contact and fixation will not be used. The plane of obliquity should be designed to allow the fragments to move in the intended direction(s) without obstructing that movement. For varus or valgus tibial deformity correction, make an oblique *coronal* plane fibula osteotomy. For rotational deformity correction as well as flexion or extension tibial

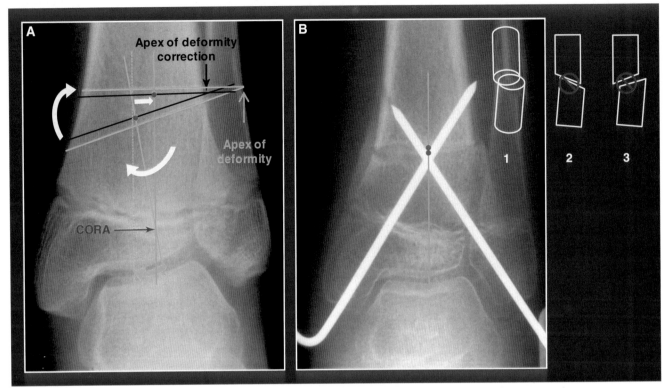

Figure 4-10. **A.** For angular deformity correction at the ankle in children, the tibial osteotomy is rarely performed at the CORA, which is usually at the growth plate, as in this case. Therefore, translation (*small yellow arrow*) in addition to angulation (*curved yellow arrows*) is required. Without translation, the axis of the distal fragment (*oblique blue line*) would be parallel with (*dotted vertical blue line*) the axis of the shaft fragment (*solid vertical blue line*), but the axes would not be colinear, as they should be. The lateral cortex of the tibia is the apex of the deformity *correction*, whereas the lateral cortex of the fibula is the apex of the deformity. **B.** A fibula osteotomy is required to enable both angulation and lateral translation of the distal fragments, and it must be made in the proper plane, in this example, the *oblique coronal plane* (*1*). The axes of the fragments have become anatomically aligned (*solid blue line*). If the osteotomy were made in the oblique sagittal plane from distal/lateral to proximal/medial (*2*), the fragments would abut each other and prevent angular deformity correction. If the osteotomy were made in the oblique sagittal plane from proximal/lateral to distal/medial (*3*), the fragments would separate and lose contact with each other, thereby possibly delaying healing.

deformity correction, make an oblique *sagittal* plane fibula osteotomy.

3. *Achieve control of the distal tibial fragment before the osteotomy is performed, if at all possible* (Figure 4-14).

After the osteotomy is performed, it is difficult (or even impossible) to appreciate the complex three-dimensional shape and alignment of the distal tibial fragment. Fixation on the "anticipated" distal fragment will make it easy to move it to the intended new location after the osteotomy is completed. It is always easy to see the shaft fragment.

4. *Cut the tibia perpendicular to the shaft for a pure rotational osteotomy* (Figure 4-15).

If the tibia is not cut perpendicular to the axis of the shaft, rotation will result in undesired flexion, extension, varus, valgus, or combinations of these deformities.

5. *For closing wedge angular deformity correction osteotomies, make the first tibial cut parallel with the ankle (while you can still see parallel), and make the second tibial cut perpendicular to the shaft on the shaft fragment* (Figure 4-16).

If the second tibial cut is not perpendicular to the axis of the shaft, any desired (or undesired) change in rotation will result in undesired flexion, extension, varus, valgus, or combinations of these deformities.

MANAGEMENT PRINCIPLE #21

Iliac crest is the ideal bone graft material for foot deformity correction surgery in children and adolescents. Allograft has advantages over autograft (Figure 4-17).

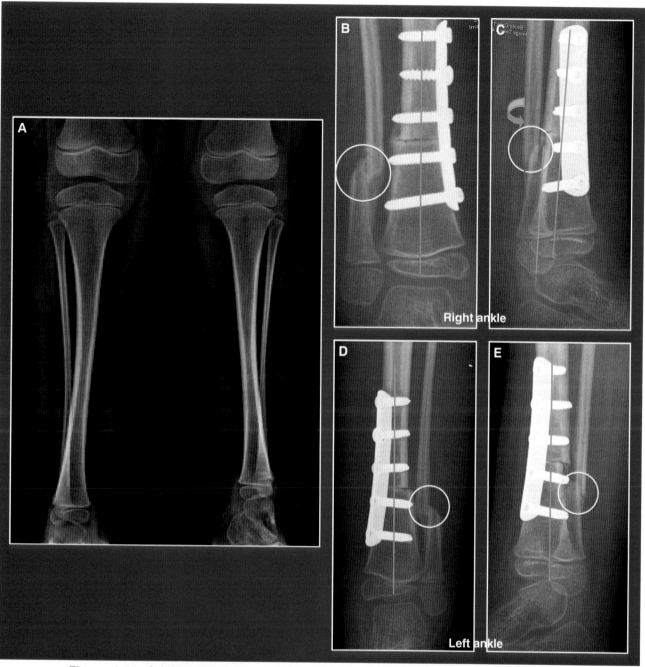

Figure 4-11. **A.** Bilateral severe external tibia and fibula rotational deformities in a child with myelomeningocele. **B.** For pure rotational deformity correction at the ankle in children, the fibula must be cut, because the central axis of rotational deformity correction is that of the tibia (*green line*). Two adjacent solid objects cannot rotate on the axis of one of them without the other resisting rotation. **C.** If a fibula osteotomy is not performed, the fibula will restrict rotation of the tibial fragments and the medial articular surface of the lateral malleolus (*purple line*) will flex or extend in relation to the lateral articular surface of the talus, thereby, creating incongruity. An *oblique sagittal plane* osteotomy of the fibula will enable the adjacent articular surfaces of the lateral malleolus and the talus to remain congruous and the axes of the distal fragments to remain parallel (*blue and green lines*) when the distal fragments are rotated around the central axis of the tibia (*green line*). **D. and E.** Forty-five degrees of rotational correction was achieved in this example. The obliquity of the fibula osteotomy ensured maintenance of some contact between the fragments (*yellow circles*) which, combined with the subperiosteal exposure of the fibula, ensured rapid healing in this extreme case of rotational deformity correction. An oblique coronal plane osteotomy of the fibula would have either created an obstruction to rotation or led to separation of the fibula fragments.

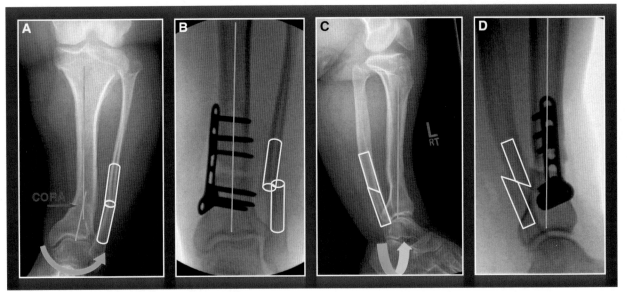

Figure 4-12. For varus and valgus correcting osteotomies, the fibula osteotomy should be made in the *oblique coronal plane*. **A.** This AP x-ray of the leg of an adolescent with achondroplasia shows the CORA in her tibia, which became the site of her varus correcting osteotomy. The fibula osteotomy was performed in the *oblique coronal plane*. **B.** The fibula osteotomy enabled frontal (coronal) plane deformity correction of the tibia at the CORA (*straight green line*). The fibula fragments slid past each other. **C.** The lateral x-ray before deformity correction with the site and direction of the fibula osteotomy indicated. **D.** The fibula osteotomy enabled coronal plane deformity correction of the tibia at the CORA (with no change in the *straight green line*). The fibula fragments slid past each other.

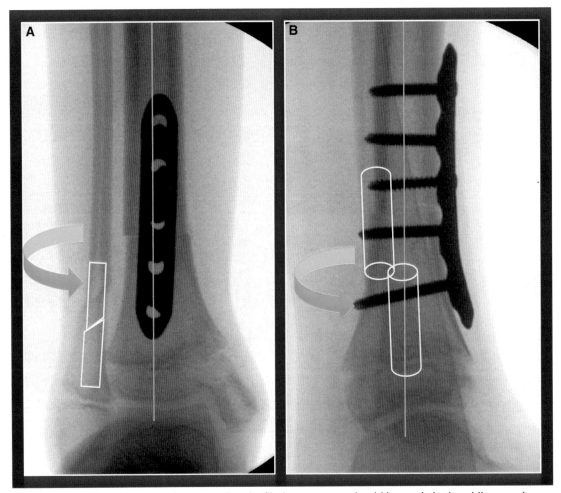

Figure 4-13. For rotational osteotomies, the fibula osteotomy should be made in the *oblique sagittal plane* **(also see Figure 4-11). A.** This AP x-ray of the ankle of a child with myelomeningocele shows the *oblique sagittal plane* of the fibula osteotomy. **B.** The lateral x-ray after rotational deformity correction shows the anterior displacement of the distal fibula fragment that enabled the tibial fragments to rotate on their common central axes.

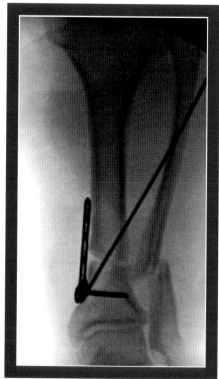

Figure 4-14. For this varus deformity correction, the plate was bent and the screws were inserted distally before the osteotomy was performed to ensure proper alignment on, and good control of, the distal fragment while the alignment of the distal fragment could still be determined. The plate and screws were then removed, the plate was straightened, the osteotomy was performed, and the plate and screws were reattached. The plate could have been attached anteriorly, thereby obviating the need to pre-bend it. For correction of a valgus deformity, pre-bending of the plate would not have been necessary regardless of where it was positioned.

The thick cortices of corticocancellous iliac crest bone grafts provide immediate structural support, and the abundant cancellous bone provides rapid early healing. We have shown that there is no difference between freeze dried iliac crest allograft and iliac crest autograft in the rate of healing, the quality of healing, and complications, based on allograft obtained from a reliable and reputable bone bank. The costs are comparable, i.e., the charge for the allograft and the surgical fee for obtaining autograft. The use of allograft obviates the time needed to obtain autograft and the need for an additional surgical site, one that is reported to be associated with significant pain. Finally, autograft is only bicortical in children and young adolescents. Allograft is tricortical, thereby making it more structurally sound and able to withstand forceful impaction into the osteotomy site.

MANAGEMENT PRINCIPLE #22

Principles of tendon transfers:

The best muscle balance across a joint exists when all of the muscles that cross the joint have normal strength. The next best muscle balance scenario exists when all of the muscles that cross a joint are equally weak or absent. The third, and

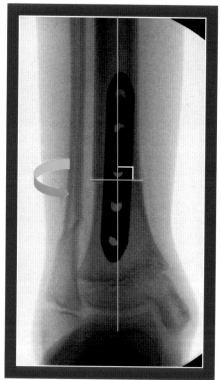

Figure 4-15. For a pure rotational osteotomy, the plate is attached distally with two screws, then removed; the osteotomy is performed perpendicular to the axis of the shaft; the plate is reattached to the distal fragment; it is then attached to the shaft with three screws after the rotational deformity has been corrected. If the osteotomy is not perpendicular to the axis of the shaft, rotation of the distal fragment will result in undesired flexion, extension, varus, valgus, or combinations of these deformities.

worst, scenario exists when there are both strong and weak muscles across a joint, as these muscle imbalances create deformities. This last scenario is typically seen in foot deformities of neuromuscular origin. It is important to improve muscle balance at the time of deformity correction; otherwise the deformities will recur. Muscle/tendon balancing is part science and part art. Attention to the following principles will improve surgical outcomes.

1. *Move the right tendon to the right location at the right tension.*

The *right muscle/tendon* unit is expendable, strong, and in phase. Moving a tendon attachment to a new location is predicated on the premise that its muscle power will no longer be needed at its original site of attachment, thereby making it expendable. The muscle should be of normal or near normal strength because, in most tendon transfers, the muscle loses strength due to a change in vector and lever arm. It is unknown whether a muscle can reliably and predictably change its phase of activity during the gait cycle based on its site of attachment. For example, it has not been shown conclusively that the posterior tibialis can change from a stance phase muscle to a swing phase muscle following transfer to the dorsum of the foot, a procedure designed to substitute for a weak anterior tibialis. It might merely act

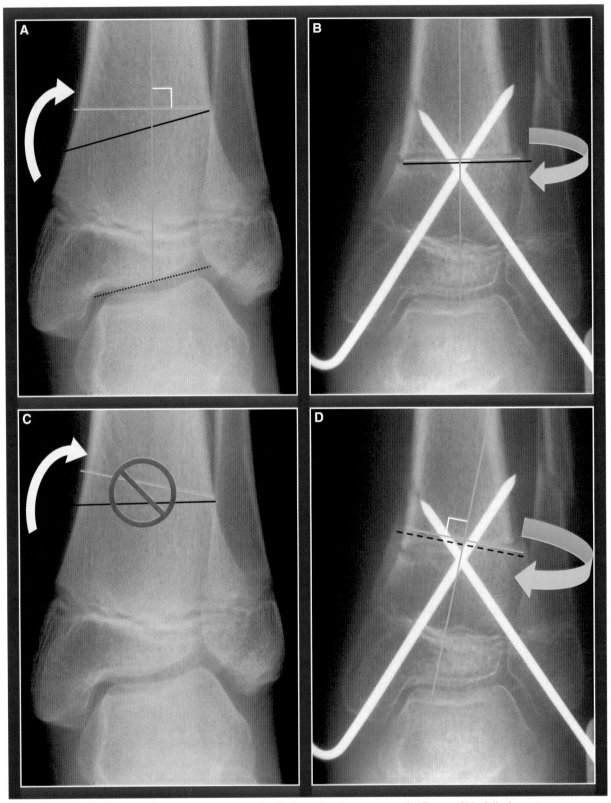

Figure 4-16. **A and B.** For a closing wedge and rotational osteotomy, the first cut (*black line*) must be the distal one and it must be parallel with the ankle joint (*black dotted line*). The second cut (*green line*) must be on the shaft fragment and it must be perpendicular to the axis of the shaft (*blue line*) or else rotation will result in undesired flexion, extension, varus, valgus, or combinations of these deformities. The crossed wires were inserted retrograde up to, but not across, the anticipated site of the distal osteotomy before the osteotomy was performed. This provided control of the distal fragment (**see Management Principle #20-3, Figure 4-14, this chapter**). The blue line is the axis of the tibia and the axis of rotation. **C and D.** If the shaft cut (*green line*) is anything other than perpendicular to the shaft, the axis of rotation is changed to a line perpendicular to that cut (*blue line*) and rotation of the distal fragment will create an undesired deformity: extension/varus with internal rotation, flexion/valgus with external rotation. The dashed black line represents the first (distal) cut in apposition with the second cut (*green line*).

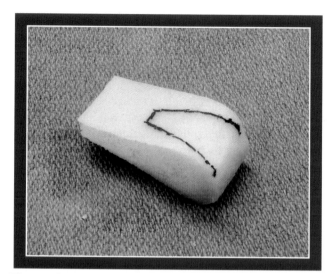

Figure 4-17. Tricortical iliac crest allograft is the ideal graft material for structural deformity correction surgery of the foot in children and adolescents.

as a tenodesis which, in some cases, could be sufficient. But, as a rule, in-phase transfers should be sought (Figure 4-18).

The *right location* for a tendon transfer is based on several factors, including the axis of motion of the joint to be crossed (which in most cases means the subtalar joint), the presence and strength of all other agonist and antagonist muscles that cross the joint, the desired anchor structure (which could be a bone or the tendon of a weak or nonfunctioning muscle), and the ease with which the tendon can directly reach the desired location without curving around structures and losing additional strength (straight vector if possible).

The *right tension* is less about science and more about art. The tension is set statically with the assumption that the desired function will follow the new form, not unlike the way a puppeteer sets tension on the strings. The foot and ankle are held in a slightly overcorrected position with firm tension set on the tendon when anchored.

2. *Tendon transfers will not correct structural deformities.*

Muscle-balancing tendon surgery will correct dynamic deformities and will likely prevent or delay the development of structural deformities (**see Management Principle #6, this chapter**). Balanced muscles will also maintain deformity correction, though perhaps for only a limited time in progressive neuromuscular disorders (**see Management Principle #7, this chapter**). Importantly, balancing muscle forces by means of tendon transfers without concurrently correcting structural deformities creates structural deformities with good muscle balance. That is not the goal (**see Management Principle #15-2, this chapter**).

3. *Tendon transfers are based on existing and anticipated patterns of muscle imbalance.*

Knowledge of the underlying condition is important. Differentiation of static vs. progressive neurologic conditions

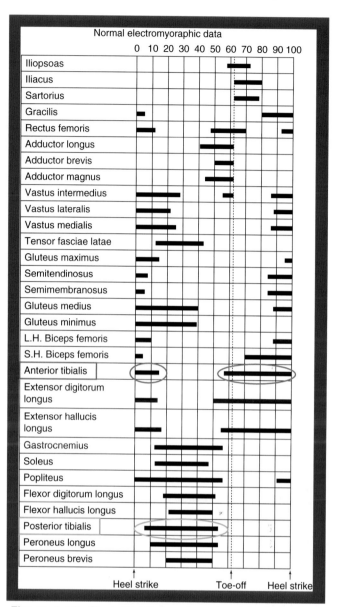

Figure 4-18. Chart of the timing of muscle activity during the gait cycle. The anterior tibialis contracts during the swing phase and at heel strike. The posterior tibialis contracts during the stance phase. It has not been shown conclusively that the phase of activity of a muscle can change if its tendon attachment site is changed.

will help determine some of the subtleties of tendon transfers and releases. Nevertheless, the rate of progression of a deformity that is due to muscle imbalance is rarely predictable. Correct the existing muscle imbalance and do your best to plan for the future.

4. *Tendon transfers are much more challenging with joint preserving reconstructions.*

But the challenge must be met. Following subtalar and triple arthrodeses, tendon transfers across the subtalar joint are of no value, because inversion and eversion motions are eliminated. The shock-absorbing function of the foot is likewise eliminated by those procedures, which is why they should be avoided (**see Management Principle #13, this chapter**).

MANAGEMENT PRINCIPLE #23

It is important to correct individual deformities in a complex multisegmental foot/ankle deformity in the proper order.

In some cases, the deformities are corrected sequentially in the same operative session, and sometimes sequential operations are required, either in close or remote proximity (Figure 4-19).

1. *Cavovarus*

Correct the *forefoot* deformity *before* the *hindfoot*. The forefoot becomes rigidly pronated (with plantar flexion of the 1st ray) before the hindfoot becomes rigidly inverted. That is the justification for performing the Coleman block test. If the forefoot is corrected before the hindfoot becomes rigidly deformed, no hindfoot deformity correction procedures are required. If the hindfoot is already rigidly deformed, it is still important to correct the forefoot first because the severity of forefoot deformity is most often greater than that of the hindfoot. Incomplete forefoot deformity correction results in the need for compensatory, rather than primary, hindfoot deformity correction procedures.

2. *Equinocavovarus*

Correct the *cavus* deformity at the *first* of two fairly closely staged operations. Correct the *equinus* at the *second* operation. This principle applies primarily to acquired deformities, though it should be considered in some congenital deformities as well.

The justification for this recommendation has to do with the number of contracted tissues at the respective sites. The contracted soft tissues in a cavus or cavovarus deformity include plantar skin, plantar fascia, short toe flexor muscles, lowest muscle belly of the abductor hallucis muscle, posterior tibial neurovascular structures, long plantar ligament, posterior tibial tendon, and the midfoot plantar joint capsules. In acquired equinus, the only significantly contracted structure is the tendo-Achilles. The only structures that can be easily released in the plantar midfoot of a cavus deformity are the plantar fascia, short toe flexors, abductor hallucis, posterior tibial tendon, and plantar capsule of the talonavicular joint. By delaying tendo-Achilles lengthening for 2 to 3 weeks, the other contracted plantar soft tissues can be stretched into dorsiflexion against the unyielding calcaneus, which is being held in position by the tendo-Achilles. Once the plantar structures are stretched, the tendo-Achilles can be lengthened with less risk of converting an equinocavus deformity into a calcaneocavus deformity.

The exception to the rule is in congenital equinocavovarus, i.e., congenital clubfoot. Cavus and equinus can be released concurrently because there are multiple posterior as well as plantar soft tissue contractures.

3. *Planovalgus*

Correct the *hindfoot* deformity *before* the *forefoot*. In contrast to the cavovarus foot, the hindfoot in a flatfoot becomes structurally deformed before the forefoot. Following hindfoot

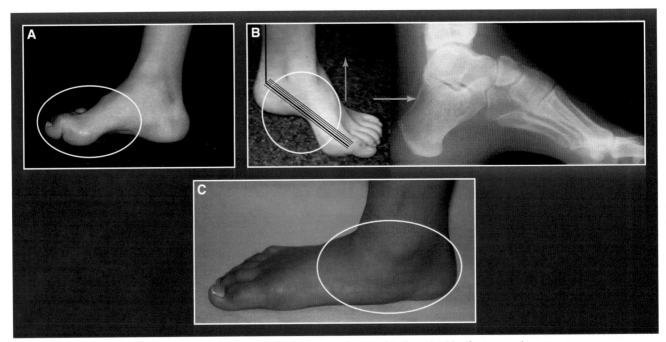

Figure 4-19. **A.** Correct the forefoot pronation (*yellow oval*) before the hindfoot varus in a cavovarus foot deformity. **B.** Correct the cavus (*yellow circle*) before the equinus in an acquired equinocavovarus foot deformity. Wait at least 2 weeks before correcting the equinus. There are multiple layers of plantar soft tissue contractures (*thin black lines*), only some of which can be released. The rest must be stretched against the calcaneus that is being held back firmly by the Achilles contracture. Concurrent release of the plantar fascia (*thick black plantar line*) and lengthening of the tendo-Achilles (*thick black posterior ankle line*) could convert an equinocavus deformity to a calcaneocavus deformity (follow the *blue arrow*). The lateral x-ray to the right of the foot image shows hyperdorsiflexion of the calcaneus with severe cavus, i.e., calcaneocavus. **C.** Correct the hindfoot valgus before the forefoot supination in a flatfoot deformity.

deformity correction with the calcaneal lengthening osteotomy, forefoot rotation is assessed intraoperatively. In most cases, particularly in younger children and adolescents, the forefoot supination deformity corrects spontaneously following hindfoot deformity correction. The plane of the metatarsal heads aligns perpendicular to the axis of the hindfoot and tibia. However, if the plane of the metatarsal heads is supinated in relation to the axis of the hindfoot and tibia following hindfoot deformity correction, a plantar flexion osteotomy of the medial cuneiform is required to correct that second structural deformity. The degree of plantar flexion is determined after the hindfoot deformity has been fully corrected.

4. *Equinoplanovalgus*

It is extremely uncommon for surgery to be required for a planovalgus deformity *without* contracture of the gastrocnemius or the entire triceps surae (tendo-Achilles). It is the heel cord contracture that usually creates the pain which is the indication for surgery. In contrast to the equinocavovarus foot, lengthening of the gastrocnemius or tendo-Achilles must be performed at the time of correction of the foot deformities.

5. *Planovalgus or cavovarus deformity with real or apparent ipsilateral tibial torsion*

External rotation of the calcaneus/acetabulum pedis is a major component of eversion, the hindfoot deformity in a planovalgus/flatfoot deformity. Internal rotation of the calcaneus/acetabulum pedis is a major component of inversion, the hindfoot deformity in a cavovarus deformity (**see Basic Principles #6 and 7, Chapter 2**). There is only one easy to document normal rotational alignment of the subtalar joint/acetabulum pedis, i.e., essentially straight alignment of the axis of the talus and the axis of the 1st metatarsal on a weight-bearing AP radiograph (average 4° abducted, range of normal 12° abducted to 10° adducted [**see Assessment Principle #18, Chapter 3**]). Assessment of tibial torsion is less precise, both clinically and radiographically. Therefore, the *inversion (internal rotation) or eversion (external rotation)* deformity of the subtalar joint should be corrected to anatomic alignment first. Then any identified residual excessive rotation of the foot in relation to the leg (positive or negative thigh–foot angle) is due to tibial torsion. Significant tibial torsion can be corrected subsequently, if necessary, during the same anesthetic or at a later date. If a tibial rotational osteotomy is inappropriately performed in an attempt to avoid correction of the hindfoot rotational deformity, the axis of flexion and extension of the ankle will become mal-oriented. This could result in abnormal stresses in the ankle that could eventually lead to premature degenerative arthritis of that joint.

If significant external tibial torsion is identified/uncovered after a flatfoot deformity has been corrected by a CLO (a rare occurrence), distal tibia and fibula internal rotation osteotomies can be performed under the same anesthetic.

If significant external tibial torsion is identified/uncovered after complex reconstruction of a cavovarus foot deformity (a very common occurrence) (**see Assessment Principle #7, Chapter 3**), distal tibia and fibula rotational osteotomies should not be performed under the same anesthetic. The tendon transfers could potentially bind down in the scar tissue and fracture callus around the osteotomies, thereby causing tethering of the tendons. If the external tibial torsion proximal to a structurally well-corrected and muscularly well-balanced foot is later noted to be a problem, isolated derotational osteotomies of the tibia and fibula can be carried out safely.

6. *Coincident subtalar joint and ankle joint valgus*

Valgus deformity can exist in the ankle joint and in the subtalar joint. The frontal plane axis of the normal ankle joint is roughly perpendicular to the tibia and parallel to the floor in weight-bearing after the age of 3 to 4 years, except in children with myelomeningocele, lipomeningocele, early onset poliomyelitis, other early onset flaccid paralytic conditions, and approximately 66% of limbs with a clubfoot (**see Assessment Principle#11, Figure 3-12, and Assessment Principle #21, Figure 3-27, Chapter 3**). This is easy to assess radiographically. There is a wide range of normal values for subtalar joint alignment from neutral to valgus. If valgus deformity exists at both levels in a symptomatic hindfoot, the *ankle valgus* should be corrected *first*. Correction is technically easy (guided growth or supramalleolar osteotomy), and there is only one easy-to-assess anatomically normal correct alignment. Once an orthogonal ankle platform is established, correction of subtalar valgus can be undertaken at the time of hardware removal, if it is still deemed necessary.

7. *Coincident subtalar joint varus and ankle joint valgus*

This combination of deformities is often seen in a recurrent/residual clubfoot and in a cavovarus foot deformity in a child with myelomeningocele. In contrast to the situation in which valgus deformity exists at both levels (**see preceding point**), the *subtalar joint* deformity should be corrected *first*. This will expose the ankle valgus deformity that can subsequently be corrected either acutely or by guided growth. The time between procedures can be considered an opportunity for valgus weight-bearing to help maintain subtalar joint deformity correction, which is sometimes a challenge for a corrected varus hindfoot.

MANAGEMENT PRINCIPLE #24

Surgical efficiency and clinical outcomes can be improved by adhering to a specific order of events during complex foot reconstruction surgery:

1. *Expose and prepare everything before completing anything.*

Many exposures are gentle and nontraumatic, but some are vigorous and forceful. Osteotomies, for example, can be forceful and could potentially disrupt an already stabilized osteotomy at another site or a tensioned tendon transfer. Release all contracted soft tissues, perform all osteotomies, and move tendons to their intended sites of attachment *before* inserting bone grafts, internally fixing osteotomies, plicating soft tissues, or tensioning tendon transfers.

2. *Perform and stabilize deformity corrections.*

The foot needs to look like a foot before tendons are tensioned. The proper tensions will be different after the deformities are corrected. Therefore, the next step is to insert bone grafts or align osteotomy surfaces and stabilize the sites with internal fixation, if needed.

3. As you proceed, close incisions that no longer need to be accessed.

This is particularly true for incisions in which there has been minimal dissection and/or minimal expectation of the need for complete hemostasis. By so doing, there will be more rapid progress to cast application after the final tendon transfer incision is closed.

4. Set proper tension on tendon lengthenings/ plications/transfers.

This is the last step, as it requires complete deformity correction for accuracy. Tendon transfers should then be performed in the order of most stable and secure to least stable and secure. An example is performing a peroneus longus to peroneus brevis transfer (using a Pulvertaft weave) before a Jones transfer.

MANAGEMENT PRINCIPLE #25

It is safe, reliable, and cosmetic to use absorbable subcuticular sutures for wound closures and no drains. Corollary: It is safe and reliable to use absorbable sutures for tendon lengthenings and transfers.

Operate carefully, but not slowly, achieving hemostasis along the way. Even complex foot reconstructions with one or more osteotomies and tendon transfers should take less than 2 hours of tourniquet time. Obtain final hemostasis after release of the tourniquet and before wound closure. It is rarely, if ever, necessary to use a drain. Use interrupted 3-0 absorbable sutures in the subcutaneous tissues and a running 4-0 absorbable subcuticular suture. Healing will be reliable and cosmetic. There is no need for cross-hatched scars. And avoiding ever having to remove sutures from children should be a professional goal and aspiration (Figure 4-20).

There are two exceptions to this principle. Nonabsorbable sutures should be used when serial casting will be required in

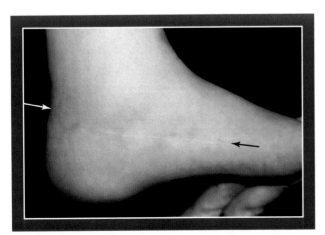

Figure 4-20. Cosmetic appearance of a healed Cincinnati incision that was used for a clubfoot operation years earlier (between the *white and black arrows*). A running 4-0 absorbable subcuticular suture was utilized.

the weeks after surgery to avoid initial excessive tension on a wound closure, as in a Cincinnati incision after a clubfoot operation in a severely deformed foot. Such a foot will have achieved full deformity correction before wound closure, but cannot assume that position after wound closure without blanching the wound edges or pulling the wound apart. The incision should be approximated with nonabsorbable vertical mattress sutures and the foot casted in mild equinovarus. The cast can be changed weekly under anesthesia and the skin stretched slowly (to avoid necrosis) until the foot assumes the fully corrected position. The final result should then be a thin cosmetic scar.

The other role for a nonabsorbable skin closure is in the first of a two-stage reconstruction, in which the second stage involves utilization of an incision created in the first stage. An example is the medial foot incision used for a plantar-medial release in a cavovarus foot deformity. It is used again 2 weeks later in the second stage for a medial cuneiform opening wedge osteotomy. A running 3-0 monofilament subcuticular suture will create less reaction and scar tissue than an absorbable suture, making it easier to close the wound in the routine fashion the second time around.

The final point regarding suture material pertains to tendon lengthenings and transfers. Absorbable sutures work quite well in both situations in children, healing reliably as long as the foot and ankle are immobilized for at least 6 weeks; 8 weeks for adolescents. Tendon weaves (Pulvertaft) heal faster and more securely than side-to-side transfers.

MANAGEMENT PRINCIPLE #26

It is safe to apply a well-padded, bivalved fiberglass cast at the end of an even complex foot reconstruction that involves multiple bone and soft tissue procedures (Figure 4-21).

Fiberglass casts should be bivalved, rather than univalved, for the best circumferential relief of pressure and accommodation of swelling. The cuts should be medial and lateral at the opposite tangents of the cylinder. The bivalved cast is overwrapped with a loosely applied elastic bandage. Excessive swelling is rarely a problem. If it occurs, it is usually within the first 24 hours postoperatively and can often be managed by slight further spreading of the anterior and posterior shells of the cast. The bivalved cast is overwrapped with fiberglass before the child is discharged from the hospital. In most cases, there should be no reason to remove the cast and examine the foot for as long as 6 weeks.

A less desirable alternative immobilization device is a bulky overpadded splint. In most cases, a splint will not hold the foot in the ideal corrected position. Therefore, it will be necessary to change the splint into a cast in the first few weeks postoperatively. It may be unnecessarily painful to change the splint into a cast in the clinic in those first few weeks and it will be unnecessarily costly to make the change in the OR.

As a general rule, bivalve the cast if an osteotomy was performed, but not if only soft tissue procedures were performed.

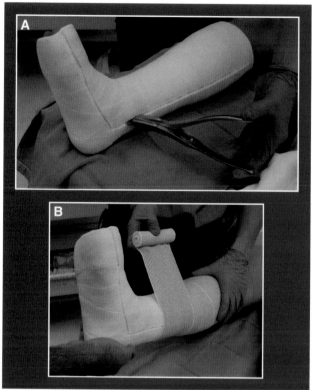

Figure 4-21. **A.** This short-leg cast was applied and immediately bivalved at the completion of a complex foot reconstruction operation that involved osteotomies and tendon transfers. **B.** The cast was loosely overwrapped with an elastic bandage. The following day, the elastic bandage was removed, the cast was overwrapped with fiberglass, and the patient was discharged from the hospital.

MANAGEMENT PRINCIPLE #27

Long-leg casts should be applied in two sections to ensure appropriate molding of the foot and protection of the soft tissues at the knee following both nonoperative and operative treatments (Figure 4-22).

The short-leg cast component is applied first, with attention focused on each of the segmental deformities of the foot. The cast is then extended above the knee after the short-leg component has hardened. It is too distracting to simultaneously focus on the position of the foot/ankle and the knee. With one-stage long-leg cast application, there is great risk that the foot molding will be inferior or that the cast padding and/or casting material will wrinkle in the popliteal fossa, creating skin ulceration. This principle applies to all long-leg casts, not just long-leg clubfoot casts.

MANAGEMENT PRINCIPLE #28

Formal physical therapy is appropriate for the successful rehabilitation of some, but not all, foot reconstructions in children and adolescents.

Children play for a living and are, therefore, their own very effective therapists. A few therapy sessions for instructions on gait retraining and strengthening are beneficial and

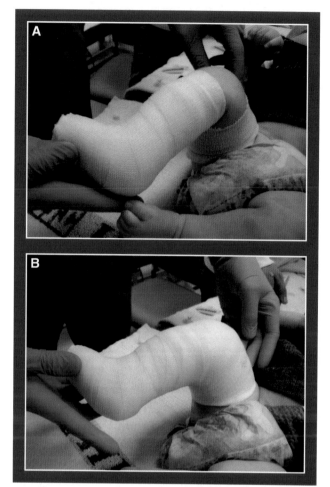

Figure 4-22. **A.** A short-leg (below the knee) cast is applied first with attention focused on the position of each of the segmental foot deformities. **B.** The cast is then extended above the 90° flexed knee. Care can be taken to ensure no bunching of the cast padding or cast material in the popliteal fossa. The appropriate thigh–foot angle can also be set.

worthwhile for some children. A good home program that is supplied by a therapist and monitored by parents is ideal.

MANAGEMENT PRINCIPLE #29

When it is not possible to make a malformed or deformed foot as comfortable and functional as a prosthesis, consider an amputation.

The technology of prosthetic design and function has advanced dramatically in the last two decades, particularly in very recent years. This has been influenced, in large part, by government-sponsored research stimulated by injuries sustained in wars abroad. Amputation, and Syme amputation in particular, is an almost routinely successful reconstructive procedure that can enable a high level of function, especially when performed early in life. Competitive sprinting, marathon running, triathlon participation, basketball, football, and other sports are all possible, even when the "disabled" athlete competes against able-bodied athletes. And the cosmetic appearance of a prosthetic can be, and usually is, better than a malformed or deformed limb, especially if the limb has undergone many operative reconstructive procedures (Figure 4-23).

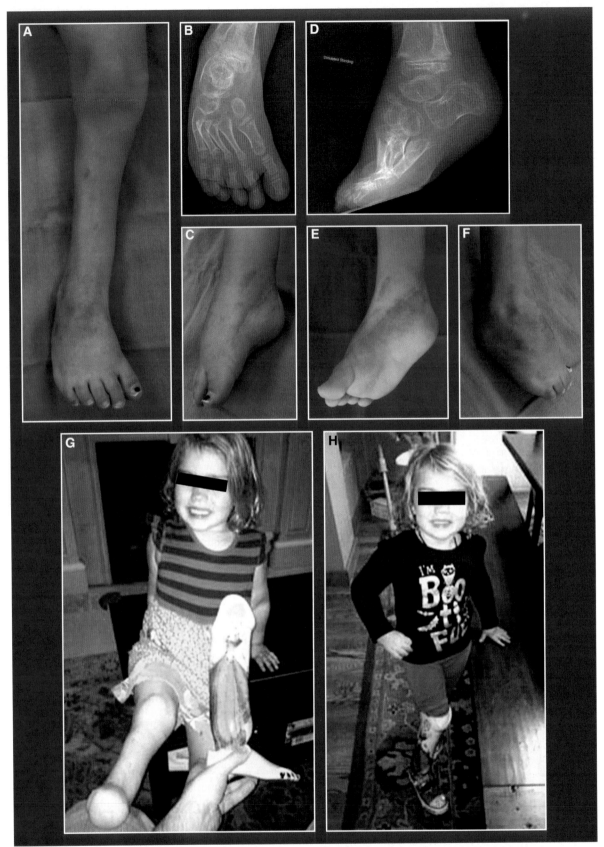

Figure 4-23. **A–F.** Completely rigid, severely deformed clubfoot in an otherwise normal, healthy 4-year-old girl. She had undergone five operative attempts by multiple surgeons to correct the deformity, including 6 months of gradual deformity correction in a three-dimensional external fixator. The deformity was overcorrected and held statically in the external fixator for several months. Following removal of the frame, the foot was casted in the overcorrected position for several weeks and then held in an AFO that she wore 23 hours per day. The deformity recurred within months after removal of the final cast, despite the use of the brace. **G and H.** Following a Syme amputation, she is now comfortable, happy, and participating in soccer, gymnastics, skiing, and other sports.

Foot and Ankle Deformities

I. ANKLE

Congenital and Acquired Short Heel Cord

1. Definition—**Deformity**
   a. Congenital or acquired contracture of the gastrocnemius or triceps surae (gastrocnemius and soleus) in an otherwise normal child with normal nerves, muscles, and bones (Figure 5-1)
   b. Acquired contracture of the gastrocnemius or triceps surae (gastrocnemius and soleus) in a child with a neuromuscular disorder
   c. Often associated with other idiopathic and acquired deformities
2. Elucidation of the segmental deformities
   a. Ankle—*plantar flexed (equinus)*
      i. Inability to dorsiflex the ankle to at least 10° above neutral with the subtalar joint held in neutral alignment (**see Assessment Principle #12, Figure 3-13, Chapter 3**)
      • If it is possible to achieve 10° of dorsiflexion with the knee flexed but not with it extended, the gastrocnemius alone is contracted.
      • If it is not possible to achieve 10° of dorsiflexion regardless of whether the knee is flexed or extended, the triceps surae (gastrocnemius and soleus) is contracted.
3. Imaging
   a. None absolutely necessary
   b. Standing anteroposterior (AP) and lateral of foot (optional)
   c. Standing AP, lateral, and mortis of ankle (optional)

4. Natural history
   a. Although never formally studied, congenital contracture of the gastrocnemius muscle or the triceps surae probably persists
   b. Acquired contractures generally increase in severity or persist at an unacceptable degree
5. Nonoperative treatment
   a. Accept it
   b. Wear high heels
   c. Twice (or more) daily heel cord stretching exercises along with nighttime dorsiflexion maintenance bracing
   d. Serial short-leg stretching casts—for children up to around 5 years of age—followed by nighttime dorsiflexion maintenance bracing
6. Operative indications
   a. Failure of nonoperative treatment to achieve and maintain at least 10° of ankle dorsiflexion above neutral with the subtalar joint in neutral alignment and the knee extended, *if* this lack of flexibility causes:
      i. pain under the metatarsal (MT) heads,
      ii. pain along the Achilles musculotendinous continuum, and/or
      iii. functional disability with gait disturbance.
7. Operative treatment with reference to the surgical techniques section of the book for each individual procedure
   a. Gastrocnemius recession (**see Chapter 7**)—*perform this* for an isolated contracture of the gastrocnemius, based on the Silverskiold test (**see Assessment Principle #12, Figure 3-13, Chapter 3**)
   b. Tendo-Achilles Lengthening (TAL) (**see four techniques in Chapter 7**)—*perform this* for contracture of

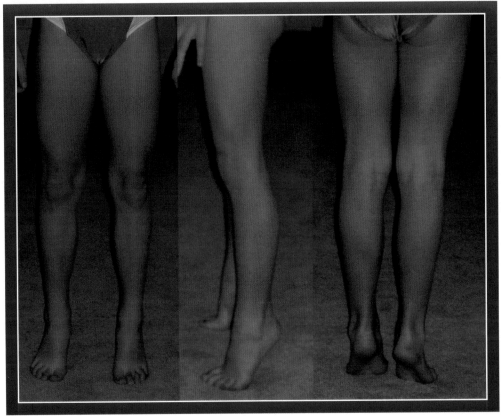

Figure 5-1. Toe-standing/walking due to congenital contracture of the gastrocnemius muscles in an otherwise normal child.

the triceps surae (gastrocnemius and soleus), based on the Silfverskiold test (**see Assessment Principle #12, Figure 3-13, Chapter 3**). The considerations for which technique to use are elucidated in **Chapter 7**.
   i. Percutaneous triple cut
   ii. Mini-open double cut slide
   iii. Open double cut slide
   iv. Open Z-lengthening

Positional Calcaneovalgus Deformity

1. Definition—**Deformity**
   a. Congenital positional hyperdorsiflexion and valgus deformity of the hindfoot (Figure 5-2A)
   b. Differential diagnosis is (Figure 5-2):
      i. Congenital vertical/oblique talus
      ii. Posteromedial tibial bowing
      iii. Paralytic calcaneus deformity
2. Elucidation of the segmental deformities
   a. Forefoot—*neutral*
   b. Midfoot—*neutral*
   c. Hindfoot—*valgus/everted or neutral*
   d. Ankle—*dorsiflexed (calcaneus)*
3. Imaging
   a. None, unless physical examination findings are equivocal

4. Natural history
   a. 100% of these correct completely without intervention
5. Nonoperative treatment
   a. None
   b. Parents can be instructed to perform daily plantar flexion stretching exercises. It might not make any difference in the rate of correction of the deformity, but it does no harm. Formal physical therapy is *not* indicated!
6. Operative indications
   a. None
7. Operative treatment with reference to the surgical techniques section of the book for each individual procedure
   a. Not applicable

Acquired Calcaneus Deformity

1. Definition—**Deformity**
   a. Calcaneus (hyperdorsiflexion) deformity of the ankle due to a weak triceps surae and a strong anterior tibialis (Figure 5-3)
   b. Due to:
      i. static muscle imbalance
         • myelomeningocele, lipomeningocele, postpoliomyelitis

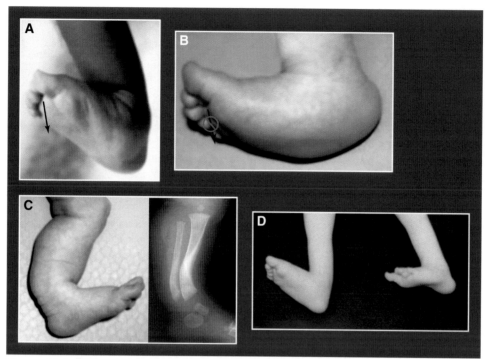

Figure 5-2. Differential diagnosis for positional calcaneovalgus deformity. **A.** Positional cal-caneovalgus. The longitudinal arch is present and the forefoot can be further plantar flexed on the hindfoot with gentle manipulation. Full passive ankle plantar flexion is not possible at birth. **B.** CVT. The longitudinal arch cannot be created by passive plantar flexion of the forefoot on the hindfoot. **C.** Posteromedial tibial bowing photo and x-ray. The deformity is actually in the tibia. The foot is well-shaped and flexible. **D.** Paralytic calcaneovalgus in a child with myelomeningocele. Weak/absent plantar flexors are noted, and there is the obvious lesion at the base of the spine.

ii. acquired muscle imbalance
  • tethered cord in myelomeningocele, lipomeningocele
iii. surgical overlengthening and/or weakening of the triceps surae, as in cerebral palsy and multiply oper-ated clubfoot

2. <u>Elucidation of the segmental deformities</u>
  a. Ankle—*dorsiflexion (calcaneus)*
3. <u>Imaging</u>
  a. Standing AP and lateral of foot (Figure 5-3)
  b. AP, lateral, and mortis of ankle

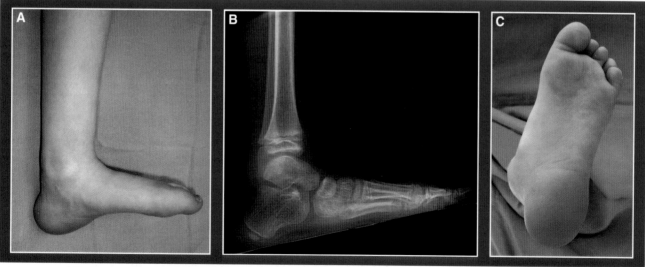

Figure 5-3. **A.** Medial view of a calcaneus foot deformity in a child with myelomeningocele. The heel pad is large, thick, and callused from excessive load-bearing. **B.** Matching lateral x-ray. **C.** Plantar view of the foot showing the large, thick, and callused heel pad, but less than normal callus formation under the MT heads.

4. Natural history
   a. Persistence of deformity, with
      i. progressive increase in callus formation on the plantar aspect of the heel
      ii. eventual fissuring of the hypertrophic and callused skin of the heel pad
      iii. ultimately, plantar heel ulceration
      iv. Pain is rarely a clinical problem because this deformity occurs most commonly in children with myelomeningocele and lipomeningocele, who have insensate skin.
   b. Progressive increase in crouched gait with gradual decrease in walking endurance. The underlying triceps surae muscle weakness, compounded by increased body weight with advancing age, leads to lever arm dysfunction (see Basic Principle #7, Figure 2-10, Chapter 2).
   c. Poor brace integrity with rapid failure of the plastic at the ankle of the ankle-foot-orthotic (AFO)

5. Nonoperative treatment
   a. Body weight reduction
   b. Increase rigidity of the AFO
6. Operative indications
   a. Failure of nonoperative attempts to maintain walking endurance and heel skin integrity
7. Operative treatment with reference to the surgical techniques section of the book for each individual procedure
   a. Anterior tibialis tendon transfer to the tendo-Achilles (see Chapter 7, Figure 7-27; Figure 5-4)

Valgus Deformity of the Ankle Joint

1. Definition—Deformity
   a. Persistence of neonatal valgus orientation of the ankle joint after age 4 to 5 years (see Assessment Principle #11, Figure 3-12, and Assessment Principle #21, Figure 3-27, Chapter 3)

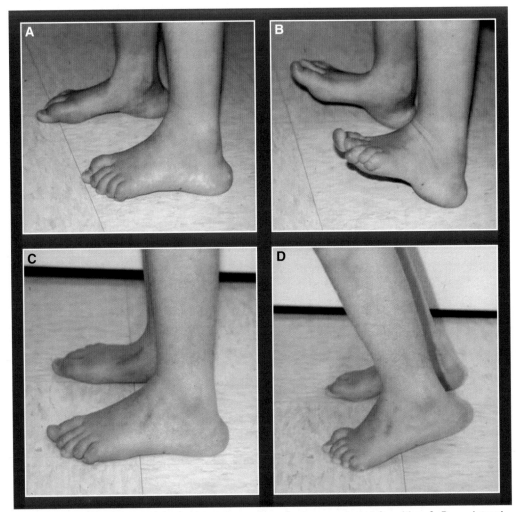

Figure 5-4. Child with L5 level myelomeningocele and calcaneus foot deformities. A. Preop lateral photos. Note the large, callused heel pads. B. She can easily heel stand, but cannot toe stand. C. One year after transfer of her anterior tibialis tendons to her tendo-Achilles, her heel pads are smaller and less callused. The peroneus tertius was released through the dorsolateral incision (not usually required). D. She was able to toe stand, though in only slightly greater than 5° of active plantar flexion. This transfer usually functions as a tenodesis that does not eliminate the need for ankle-foot orthoses, but it improves or eliminates the crouched gait and increases the useful life of the AFOs.

2. Elucidation of the segmental deformities
   a. Ankle—*valgus*
      i. Greater than 4° of valgus orientation of the articular surface of the distal tibia compared with the axis of the tibial shaft after the age of 4 to 5 years
3. Imaging
   a. AP, lateral, and mortis of the ankle (**see Assessment Principle #21, Figure 3-27, Chapter 3**)
4. Natural history
   a. Valgus orientation of the ankle joint is *normal* from birth (actually, from the time of in utero joint formation at 7 to 9 weeks' gestation) until approximately age 4 to 5 years. The valgus alignment gradually corrects to neutral by that age in most normal children.
   b. Valgus orientation of the ankle joint is reclassified as a *deformity* if it persists after approximately age 4 to 5 years
      i. The average lateral distal tibia angle (LDTA) after age 4 to 5 years is 89° (1° of valgus), with the normal range of 86° to 92° (4° of valgus to 2° of varus); therefore, >4° of valgus is abnormal.
   c. Congenital valgus orientation of the ankle joint *persists* as a *deformity* in:
      i. up to 66% of limbs with clubfoot deformity
      ii. fibula hemimelia, often as a ball-and-socket joint
      iii. essentially all limbs affected by myelomeningocele, lipomeningocele, poliomyelitis, spinal cord tumor or injury, and other lower extremity paralyzing conditions (not cerebral palsy) that affect young children
   d. Valgus *deformity* of the ankle *can develop* following:
      i. injury to the lateral distal tibial physis and/or distal fibula physis
      ii. fibula pseudarthrosis in congenital anterolateral bowing of the tibia and fibula, with or without tibial pseudarthrosis and with or without neurofibromatosis
   e. Persistent and developmental valgus deformities of the ankle joint can cause:
      i. lateral ankle/hindfoot pain from impingement of the lateral malleolus, peroneal tendons, and calcaneus
      ii. medial ankle/hindfoot pain from stretch of the medial ankle joint and subtalar joint ligaments
      iii. plantar–medial heel pain due to excessive loading on that area of the heel pad
      iv. skin pressure irritation and/or pain under the medial malleolus due to weight-bearing on the firm shoe counter or on the hard plastic of an AFO (in children with paralytic conditions)
5. Nonoperative treatment
   a. None indicated for asymptomatic cases
   b. Over-the-counter, cushioned, semirigid arch supports (Figure 5-31) to invert the neutral subtalar joint into varus to compensate for the valgus deformity of the ankle joint. These are *contraindicated* if the gastrocnemius or entire triceps surae is contracted.
   c. Adjust or modify the padding in an AFO in a child with an underlying paralytic condition

6. Operative indications
   a. Failure of nonoperative treatment to relieve the:
      i. lateral ankle/hindfoot pain from impingement of the lateral malleolus, peroneal tendons, and calcaneus
      ii. medial ankle/hindfoot pain from stretch of the medial ankle joint and subtalar joint ligaments
      iii. skin pressure irritation and/or pain under the medial malleolus due to weight-bearing on the shoe counter or the hard plastic of an AFO (in a child with an underlying paralytic condition)
   b. Progressive valgus deformity due to injury to the lateral distal tibial physis and/or distal fibula physis
7. Operative treatment with reference to the surgical techniques section of the book for each individual procedure
   a. Medial distal tibia guided growth with retrograde medial malleolus screw (**see Chapter 8**)—*perform this* in a skeletally immature child
   b. Distal tibia and fibula valgus-correction osteotomies (**see Management Principle #20, Figures 4-10 and 4-12, Chapter 4**), (**see Chapter 8**)—*perform this* in a skeletally mature adolescent
   c. Resection and fat grafting of the physeal bar (if appropriate) with or without concurrent distal tibia and fibula valgus-correction osteotomies (**see Chapter 8**)—*perform this* in a skeletally immature child with a small physeal bar
   d. Completion of the distal tibial and fibula growth arrests (epiphysiodeses) with concurrent distal tibia and fibula valgus-correction osteotomies (**see Chapter 8**)—*perform this* in a skeletally immature child with a large, irresectable physeal bar

Valgus Deformity of the Ankle Joint *and* the Hindfoot

1. Definition—**Deformities**
   a. Valgus orientation of the ankle joint after age 4 to 5 years (**see Assessment Principle #11, Figure 3-12, and Assessment Principle #21, Figure 3-27, Chapter 3**) *and*
   b. Valgus deformity of the hindfoot, with or without eversion of the subtalar joint, as seen in:
      i. Idiopathic flatfoot
      ii. Congenital vertical talus (CVT)
      iii. Congenital oblique talus (COT)
      iv. Skewfoot
      v. Tarsal coalition
      vi. Congenital talocalcaneal synostosis associated with
         • fibula hemimelia
         • tibial hemimelia
         • lower extremity hemiatrophy
         • other syndromes and chromosome abnormalities
      vii. Overcorrected clubfoot
         • translational
         • rotational
2. Elucidation of the segmental deformities
   a. Hindfoot—*valgus* or *valgus/eversion*

b. Ankle—*valgus*

   i. Greater than 4° of valgus orientation of the articular surface of the distal tibia compared with the axis of the tibial shaft after the age of 4 to 5 years

3. Imaging

   a. Standing AP, lateral, and Harris axial views of the foot (**see Assessment Principle #18, Figures 3-20, and 3-24, Chapter 3**)

   b. AP, lateral, and mortis of the ankle (**see Assessment Principle #21, Figure 3-27, Chapter 3**)

4. Natural history

   a. *Valgus* orientation of the *ankle joint* is normal from birth (actually, from the time of in utero joint formation at 7 to 9 weeks' gestation) until approximately age 4 to 5 years. The valgus alignment gradually corrects to neutral by that age in most normal children.

      i. Valgus orientation of the ankle joint is reclassified as a *deformity* if it persists after approximately age 4 to 5 years

         • The average LDTA after age 4 to 5 years is 89° (1° of valgus), with the normal range of 86° to 92° (4° of valgus to 2° of varus); therefore, >4° of valgus is abnormal.

      ii. Congenital valgus orientation of the ankle joint *persists* as a *deformity* in:

         • up to 66% of limbs with clubfoot deformity

         • fibula hemimelia, often as a ball-and-socket joint

         • essentially all limbs affected by myelomeningocele, lipomeningocele, poliomyelitis, spinal cord tumor or injury, and other lower extremity paralyzing conditions (not cerebral palsy) that affect young children

      iii. Valgus *deformity* of the ankle *can develop* following:

         • injury to the lateral distal tibial physis and/or distal fibula physis

         • fibula pseudarthrosis in congenital anterolateral bowing of the tibia and fibula, with or without tibial pseudarthrosis and with or without neurofibromatosis

      iv. Persistent and developmental valgus deformities of the ankle joint can cause:

         • lateral ankle/hindfoot pain from impingement of the lateral malleolus, peroneal tendons, and calcaneus

         • medial ankle/hindfoot pain from stretch of the medial ankle joint and subtalar joint ligaments

         • plantar–medial heel pain due to excessive loading on that area of the heel pad

         • skin pressure irritation and/or pain under the medial malleolus due to weight-bearing on the firm shoe counter or on the hard plastic of an AFO (in children with paralytic conditions)

   b. *Valgus* deformity of the *hindfoot*, with or without eversion of the subtalar joint, can cause axial loading pain under the head of the talus and/or impingement-type pain in the sinus tarsi area

5. Nonoperative treatment

   a. None indicated for asymptomatic cases

   b. Over-the-counter, cushioned, semirigid arch supports (Figure 5-31) to invert the subtalar joint into varus to correct the subtalar valgus and to attempt to compensate for the valgus deformity of the ankle joint. These are *contraindicated* if the gastrocnemius or entire triceps surae is contracted.

   c. Adjust or modify the padding in an AFO in a child with an underlying paralytic condition

6. Operative indications

   a. Failure of nonoperative treatment to relieve the:

      i. lateral ankle/hindfoot pain from impingement of the lateral malleolus, peroneal tendons, and calcaneus

      ii. medial ankle/hindfoot pain from stretch of the medial ankle joint and subtalar joint ligaments

      iii. skin pressure irritation and/or pain under the medial malleolus due to weight-bearing on the shoe counter or the hard plastic of an AFO (in a child with an underlying paralytic condition)

      iv. axial loading pain under the head of the talus and/or impingement-type pain in the sinus tarsi area

   b. Progressive valgus deformity due to injury to the lateral distal tibial physis and/or distal fibula physis

7. Operative treatment with reference to the surgical techniques section of the book for each individual procedure

   a. Correct the ankle valgus *first*. There is only one, easy-to-assess, stable anatomic alignment of the ankle joint (**see Management Principle #23-6, Chapter 4**).

      i. Medial distal tibia guided growth with retrograde medial malleolus screw (**see Chapter 8**)—*perform this* in a skeletally immature child

      ii. Distal tibia and fibula valgus-correction osteotomies (**see Chapter 8**)—*perform this* in a skeletally mature adolescent

      iii. Resection and fat grafting of the physeal bar (if appropriate) with or without concurrent distal tibia and fibula valgus-correction osteotomies (**see Chapter 8**)—*perform this* in a skeletally immature child with a small physeal bar

      iv. Completion of the distal tibial and fibula growth arrests (epiphysiodeses) with concurrent distal tibia and fibula valgus-correction osteotomies (**see Chapter 8**)—*perform this* in a skeletally immature child with a large, irresectable physeal bar

   b. Once the ankle joint is anatomically aligned, correct the subtalar joint valgus according to the type of valgus present

      i. Idiopathic flatfoot—calcaneal lengthening osteotomy (**see Chapter 8**)

      ii. CVT (in the older child)—naviculectomy (**see Chapter 8**)

      iii. COT (in the older child)—calcaneal lengthening osteotomy (**see Chapter 8**)

      iv. Skewfoot—calcaneal lengthening osteotomy (**see Chapter 8**)

      v. Tarsal coalition—calcaneal lengthening osteotomy (**see Chapter 8**)

vi. Congenital talocalcaneal valgus synostosis associated with fibula hemimelia, tibial hemimelia, lower extremity hemiatrophy, other syndromes and chromosome abnormalities—posterior calcaneus displacement osteotomy (**see Chapter 8**)

vii. Overcorrected clubfoot
- Translational—posterior calcaneus displacement osteotomy (**see Chapter 8**)
- Rotational—calcaneal lengthening osteotomy (**see Chapter 8**)

II. CAVUS

Cavovarus Foot (*Excluding* Those Due to Cerebral Palsy—See Below)

1. <u>Definition</u>—**Deformity**
   a. Acquired and usually progressive pronation deformity of the forefoot on the hindfoot that creates cavus deformity of the medial midfoot. There is secondary acquired and usually progressive varus/inversion deformity of the hindfoot. The ankle can be in dorsiflexion, plantar flexion, or neutral. It is the manifestation of a neuromuscular disorder, rather than a primary deformity, unless proven otherwise (Figure 5-5).

2. <u>Elucidation of the segmental deformities</u>
   a. Forefoot—*pronated*
   b. Midfoot—*adducted* or *neutral*
   c. Hindfoot—*varus/inverted*
   d. Ankle—*plantar flexed, neutral,* or *dorsiflexed*
      i. *NOTE:* It is *uncommon* for there to be contracture of the tendo-Achilles or the gastrocnemius in a cavovarus foot in a child with Charcot–Marie–Tooth (CMT) disease. The apparent ankle equinus (plantar flexion of the foot at the ankle) is, in fact, usually forefoot equinus, i.e., cavus (plantar flexion of the forefoot on the hindfoot) (**see Assessment Principle #12, Figure 3-14, Chapter 3**). The ankle is often hyperdorsiflexed with an exaggerated calcaneal pitch.
   e. Tibia—*external torsion*
      i. In most children with cavovarus foot deformities, regardless of the etiologic underlying neuromuscular

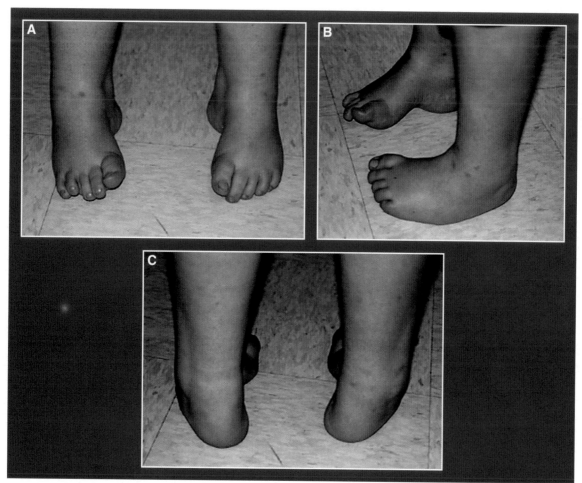

Figure 5-5. Cavovarus foot deformities in a young boy with CMT disease. **A.** Top/front view shows cavus with varus heels, visible medially. **B.** Side views show cavus of right foot and adductus of left foot. **C.** Posterior view shows varus heels and forefoot adductus.

disorder, there is coincident external tibial torsion (**see Assessment Principle #7, Chapter 3**).

  f. Muscle imbalances (*opposite* those seen in dorsal bunion deformities) (Figure 5-6)

    i. Weak anterior tibialis

    ii. Strong peroneus longus

    iii. Recruited and, therefore, stronger extensor hallucis longus (EHL) than flexor hallucis longus (FHL)

  g. "Flexibility" classification for the forefoot and hindfoot (unpublished)

    i. *Flexible* =

      • dynamic deformity of the *forefoot* or *hindfoot* that corrects with tendon transfers

      • dynamic and flexible deformity of the *hindfoot* that corrects following correction of the forefoot deformity and with tendon transfers

    ii. *Stiff* = structural deformity of the forefoot or hindfoot that corrects with soft tissue releases

    iii. *Rigid* = structural deformity of the forefoot or hindfoot that requires osteotomies and/or arthrodeses

  h. *Cavovarus Flexibility Classification System* (Forefoot-Hindfoot) (unpublished)

    i. Flexible–Flexible

    ii. Stiff–Flexible

    iii. Rigid–Flexible

    iv. Rigid–Stiff

    v. Rigid–Rigid

    vi. Late Rigid–Rigid

3. Imaging

  a. Standing AP and lateral of foot (**see Assessment Principle #18, Figures 3-20 and 3-22, Chapter 3**)

  b. Standing AP block x-ray with 2.5-cm block under lateral forefoot (4th and 5th MT heads) (**see Assessment Principle #19, Figure 3-24, Chapter 3**)

  c. Standing AP, lateral, and mortis of ankle

  d. Standing AP and lateral thoracolumbar spine

  e. AP pelvis (in patients with CMT or suspected CMT)

4. Natural history

  a. Progressive increase in the severity and rigidity of the segmental deformities with pain, gait instability, and

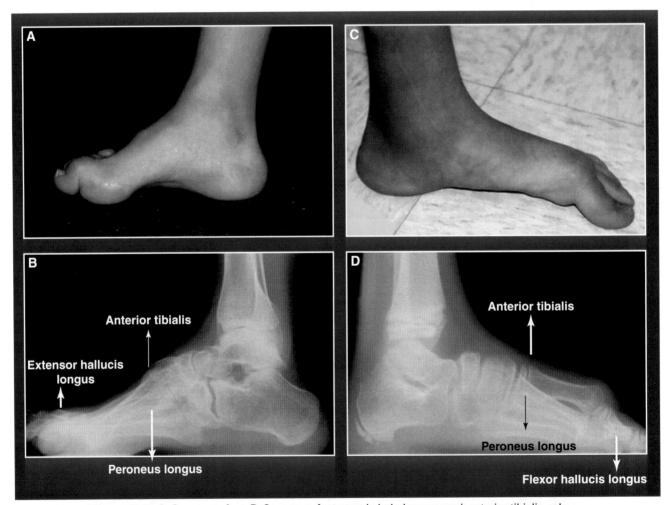

Figure 5-6. A. Cavovarus foot. **B.** Cavovarus foot muscle imbalances: weak anterior tibialis, relatively stronger peroneus longus, recruited extensor hallucis longus to compensate for weak anterior tibialis. **C.** Dorsal bunion deformity. **D.** Dorsal bunion muscle imbalances: strong anterior tibialis, weak peroneus longus, recruited FHL to compensate for weak peroneus longus.

skin pressure injuries (inflammation, callus formation, blistering, ulceration) under the 1st and 5th MT heads and at the base of the 5th MT (**see Assessment Principle #9, Figure 3-5, Chapter 3**).

5. <u>Nonoperative treatment</u>
   a. Accommodative shoe wear with over-the-counter soft arch supports *pending results* of neuromuscular workup—then operate.

6. <u>Operative indications</u>
   a. Pain, gait instability, skin pressure injuries, and/or progressive deformity
      i. *following* completion of a neuromuscular workup, with treatment of the underlying condition if treatment exists

7. <u>Operative treatment</u>, based on the *Cavovarus Flexibility Classification System*, with reference to the surgical techniques section of the book for each individual procedure (**see Management Principles #13, 15, 16, 22, 23-1, and 24, Chapter 4**). NOTE: If a gastrocnemius recession or a tendo-Achilles lengthening is needed, it should be performed in the second stage of a 2-stage procedure (**see Management Principle #23-2, Chapter 4**).
   a. Flexible–Flexible
      i. Peroneus longus to peroneus brevis transfer (**see Chapter 7**)
      ii. Posterior tibialis tendon lengthening—Z-lengthening or intramuscular recession (**see Chapter 7**)
   b. Stiff–Flexible
      i. Superficial plantar-medial release (**see Chapter 7**)
      ii. Posterior tibialis tendon lengthening—Z-lengthening or intramuscular recession (**see Chapter 7**)
      iii. Peroneus longus to peroneus brevis transfer (**see Chapter 7**)
      iv. Percutaneous tenotomy of FHL and FDL to toes 2 to 5 (**see Chapter 7**)
   c. Rigid–Flexible
      i. *Stage 1*
         • Superficial plantar-medial release (**see Chapter 7**)
         • Posterior tibialis tendon lengthening—Z-lengthening or intramuscular recession (**see Chapter 7**)
         • Percutaneous tenotomy of FHL and FDL to toes 2 to 5 (**see Chapter 7**)
      ii. *Stage 2—2 weeks later*
         • Medial cuneiform (dorsiflexion) plantar-based opening wedge osteotomy (**see Chapter 8**)
         • Peroneus longus to peroneus brevis transfer (**see Chapter 7**)
         • *Possible* posterior calcaneus lateral displacement osteotomy (**see Chapter 8**)
         • *Possible* split anterior tibialis tendon transfer (**see Chapter 7**)
         • *Possible* Jones transfer of extensor hallux longus to 1st MT neck with hallux interphalangeal (IP) joint tenodesis (**see Chapter 7**) or arthrodesis (**see Chapter 8**)
         • *Possible* Hibbs transfer of extensor digitorum communis to peroneus tertius or cuboid (**see Chapter 7**)
   d. Rigid–Stiff
      i. *Stage 1*
         • Deep plantar-medial release (**see Chapter 7**)
         • Percutaneous tenotomy of FHL and FDL to toes 2 to 5 (**see Chapter 7**)
      ii. *Stage 2—2 weeks later*
         • Medial cuneiform (dorsiflexion) plantar-based opening wedge osteotomy (**see Chapter 8**)
         • Peroneus longus to peroneus brevis transfer (**see Chapter 7**)
         • *Possible* posterior calcaneus lateral displacement osteotomy (**see Chapter 8**)
         • *Possible* split anterior tibialis tendon transfer (**see Chapter 7**)
         • *Possible* Jones transfer of extensor hallux longus to 1st MT neck with hallux IP joint tenodesis (**see Chapter 7**) or arthrodesis (**see Chapter 8**)
         • *Possible* Hibbs transfer of extensor digitorum communis to peroneus tertius or cuboid (**see Chapter 7**)
   e. Rigid–Rigid
      i. *Stage 1*
         • Deep plantar-medial release (**see Chapter 7**)
         • Percutaneous tenotomy of FHL and FDL to toes 2 to 5 (**see Chapter 7**)
      ii. *Stage 2—2 weeks later*
         • Medial cuneiform (dorsiflexion) plantar-based opening wedge osteotomy (**see Chapter 8**)
         • Peroneus longus to peroneus brevis transfer (**see Chapter 7**)
         • Posterior calcaneus lateral displacement osteotomy (**see Chapter 8**)
         • *Possible* split anterior tibialis tendon transfer (**see Chapter 7**)
         • *Possible* Jones transfer of extensor hallux longus to 1st MT neck with hallux IP joint tenodesis (**see Chapter 7**) or arthrodesis (**see Chapter 8**)
         • *Possible* Hibbs transfer of extensor digitorum communis to peroneus tertius or cuboid (**see Chapter 7**)
   f. Late Rigid–Rigid
      i. *Stage 1*
         • Deep plantar-medial release (**see Chapter 7**)
         • Percutaneous tenotomy of FHL and FDL to toes 2 to 5 (**see Chapter 7**)
      ii. *Stage 2—2 weeks later or concurrent*
         • Midfoot wedge resection/arthrodesis (**see Chapter 8**)
            • or, Triple arthrodesis (**see Chapter 8 and Management Principle #13, Chapter 4**)
         • *Possible* split anterior tibialis tendon transfer (**see Chapter 7**)
         • *Possible* Jones transfer of extensor hallux longus to 1st MT neck with hallux IP joint tenodesis (**see Chapter 7**) or arthrodesis (**see Chapter 8**)
         • *Possible* Hibbs transfer of extensor digitorum communis to peroneus tertius or cuboid (**see Chapter 7**)

- *Possible* posterior tibialis tendon transfer through the interosseous membrane to the dorsum of the foot. *Best indication* is a strong posterior tibialis and no other functional muscle power (**see Chapter 7**)

Cavovarus Foot (Due to Cerebral Palsy)

1. Definition – **Deformity**
   a. Acquired and progressive varus deformity of the hindfoot with secondary pronation of the forefoot on the hindfoot creating a cavus midfoot deformity. The ankle is plantar flexed, because there is always associated contracture of the gastrocnemius or the entire triceps surae. The deformities are the result of muscle imbalances due to the cerebral injury rather than being primary deformities. Cavovarus is most commonly seen in children with spastic hemiplegia (Figure 5-7).
2. Elucidation of the segmental deformities
   a. Forefoot—*pronated*
   b. Midfoot—*adducted* or *neutral*
   c. Hindfoot—*varus/inverted*
   d. Ankle—*plantar flexed (equinus)*

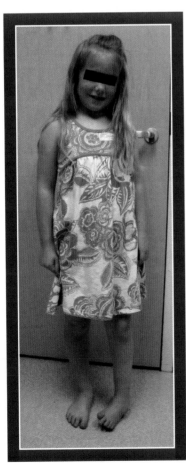

Figure 5-7. An 8-year-old girl with left hemiplegic cerebral palsy and with an equinocavovarus foot deformity.

e. Tibia—*external torsion.*
   i. In most children with cavovarus foot deformities, including those with cerebral palsy, there is coincident external tibial torsion (**see Assessment Principle #7, Chapter 3**).
f. Muscle imbalances
   i. Greater spasticity in the anterior tibialis and posterior tibialis than in the peroneal muscles
   ii. Occasionally, the peroneus longus is overpowering the anterior tibialis
3. Imaging
   a. Standing AP and lateral of foot (**see Assessment Principle #18, Figures 3-20 and 3-22**)
   b. Standing AP block x-ray is *not* reliable in children with cerebral palsy, because the spastic inverters often do not relax sufficiently to allow the subtalar joint to evert (to reveal the true flexibility of the subtalar joint)
   c. Standing AP, lateral, and mortis of ankle
4. Natural history
   a. Progressive increase in the severity and rigidity of the segmental deformities with pain, gait instability, and skin pressure injuries (inflammation, callus formation, blistering, ulceration) at the base of the 5th MT, over the dorsolateral aspect of the talar head in the sinus tarsi region (related to rubbing in the AFO), and occasionally under the 1st MT head
5. Nonoperative treatment
   a. Physical therapy—stretching
   b. Bracing—AFO
   c. Injection of botulinum toxin (BOTOX) into the most spastic muscles
   d. Serial below-the-knee (short-leg) stretching casts
   e. Tone-reducing medications, such as baclofen
6. Operative indications
   a. Pain, gait instability, skin pressure injuries, and/or progressive deformity that are not controlled with nonoperative modalities
   i. Ideally, in children over the age of 6 to 7 years
7. Operative treatment with reference to the surgical techniques section of the book for each individual procedure
   a. Rancho procedure
   i. Split anterior tibialis tendon transfer (**see Chapter 7**)
   ii. Posterior tibialis tendon lengthening
   iii. Strayer gastrocnemius recession (**see Chapter 7**)
   - Rarely, if ever, a tendo-Achilles lengthening. The soleus is rarely contracted in children with cerebral palsy, and so a TAL should not be necessary. Overlengthening the tendo-Achilles results in a decrease/weakening of the ground reaction force and leads to lever arm dysfunction with an increased crouched gait (**see Basic Principle #7, Figure 2-10, Chapter 2**).
   b. If rigid, severe forefoot pronation and hindfoot varus exist, those deformities must be corrected (**see Management Principles #15, 16, and 22-2, Chapter 4**) concurrent with muscle balancing procedures, as the latter will

not correct the former (**see Management Principles #15 and 22-2, Chapter 4**).

    i. If the hindfoot varus is *flexible*: superficial plantar-medial release (S-PMR) (**see Chapter 7**) plus posterior tibialis tendon lengthening—Z-lengthening or intramuscular recession (**see Chapter 7**)

    ii. If the hindfoot varus is *not* flexible: Deep plantar-medial release (D-PMR) (**see Chapter 7**)

    iii. If rigid forefoot pronation persists after S-PMR or D-PMR:

- Medial cuneiform (dorsiflexion) plantar-based opening wedge osteotomy (**see Chapter 8**)
- Peroneus longus to peroneus brevis transfer (**see Chapter 7**) rather than a split anterior tibialis tendon transfer, as the latter will potentiate the forefoot pronation in the face of a strong peroneus longus

Calcaneocavus (Transtarsal Cavus) Foot

1. <u>Definition</u>—**Deformity**
   a. Plantar flexion of the entire forefoot on the hindfoot with hyperdorsiflexion of the hindfoot
      i. due to muscle imbalance with weakness of the triceps surae, but preservation of strength in the posterior tibialis and peroneal muscles
      ii. seen in some children with myelomeningocele, postpoliomyelitis, and other paralytic conditions (Figure 5-8)
2. <u>Elucidation of the segmental deformities</u>
   a. Forefoot—*plantar flexed*
      i. plantar flexion of the entire forefoot on the hindfoot, creating a transtarsal cavus
      ii. MTs are parallel with each other in the sagittal plane.
   b. Midfoot—*neutral*
   c. Hindfoot—usually *neutral* with exaggerated calcaneal pitch
   d. Ankle
      i. *Dorsiflexed*
      ii. often, *valgus* orientation
3. <u>Imaging</u>
   a. Standing AP and lateral of foot
   b. Standing AP, lateral, and mortis of ankle
   c. Standing AP and lateral thoracolumbar spine
4. <u>Natural history</u>
   a. Progressive increase in the severity and rigidity of the cavus deformity with increasing crouched gait along with pain and skin pressure injuries (inflammation, callus formation, blistering, ulceration) under the calcaneus and the MT heads as the weight-bearing pressures are concentrated under a progressively smaller plantar surface area
5. <u>Nonoperative treatment</u>
   a. Tall arch support
6. <u>Operative indications</u>
   a. Pain under the heel and/or the MT heads with weight-bearing (if the skin is sensate)

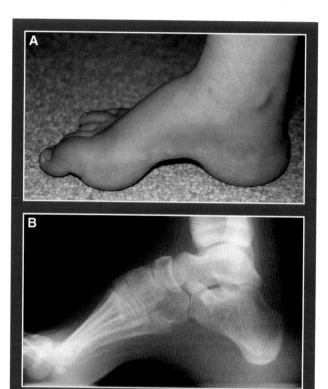

Figure 5-8. Calcaneocavus foot deformity in a teenager with S1 level myelomeningocele. **A.** Medial photo of foot shows exaggerated arch height across the entire midfoot. Though not visible in this photo, the hindfoot/subtalar joint is in neutral alignment. The soft tissues under the MT heads and the calcaneus are thick and callused. **B.** Standing lateral radiograph shows transtarsal cavus with relative parallelism of all MTs. In a cavovarus foot by contrast, the 1st MT would be hyperplantar flexed in relation to the 5th MT (Figure 3-25). The calcaneus, in this foot, is hyperdorsiflexed.

    b. Ulceration, or skin at risk of ulceration, under the heel and/or the MT heads (if the skin is insensate)

7. <u>Operative treatment</u> with reference to the surgical techniques section of the book for each individual procedure
   a. Posterior calcaneus dorsal and posterior displacement osteotomy (**see Chapter 8**)
      i. with plantar fasciotomy (**see Chapter 7**)
      ii. with possible anterior tibialis tendon lengthening
   b. Midfoot wedge resection/arthrodesis—*perform this* for the most severe and rigid cases (**see Chapter 8**)

III. CLUBFOOT

Congenital Clubfoot (Talipes Equinovarus)

1. <u>Definition</u>—**Deformity**
   a. Congenital cavus, adductus, varus, and equinus deformities that are not passively correctable (Figure 5-9)
   b. Most are idiopathic, though some are associated with myelomeningocele, arthrogryposis, and other syndromes and disorders.

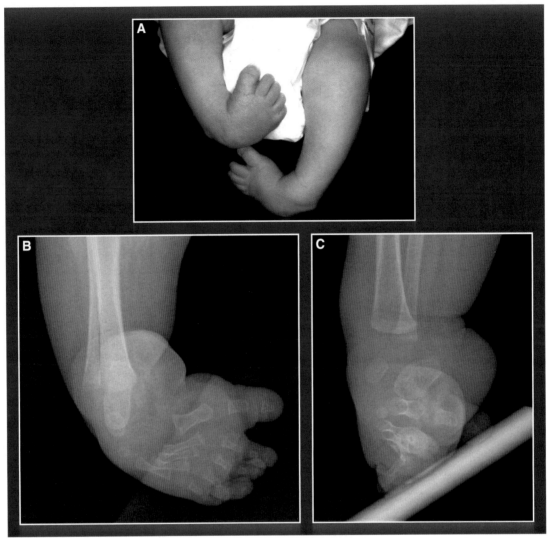

Figure 5-9. **A.** An infant with congenital clubfeet with the obvious deformities of cavus, adductus, varus/inversion, and equinus. (From Mosca VS. The Foot. In: Morrissy RT, Weinstein SL, eds. *Lovell and Winter's Pediatric Orthopaedics.* 5th ed. Philadelphia, PA: Lippincott Williams & Wilkins; 2001:1153, Figure 29-1.) **B.** AP radiograph shows the severe inversion and adductus. **C.** Lateral radiograph shows the severe equinus, cavus, and adductus. The hindfoot is pointing to the left and the forefoot is pointing to the right.

2. Elucidation of the segmental deformities
   a. Forefoot—*pronated*
   b. Midfoot—*adducted*
   c. Hindfoot—*varus/inverted*
   d. Ankle—*plantar flexed (equinus)*
3. Imaging
   a. Not necessary for diagnosis
   b. Maximum dorsiflexion/abduction/eversion AP and lateral of foot (**see Figure 5-9**)—indicated to:
      i. confirm residual deformities preoperatively after failing nonoperative treatment
      ii. confirm apparent or obvious recurrent deformities after nonoperative or operative treatment, particularly when contemplating further nonoperative or operative treatment
      iii. confirm deformity correction following operative treatment

c. Hip screening imaging for idiopathic clubfoot is *not* indicated—no documented association of the two deformities
4. Natural history
   a. Persistence of deformity with pain, functional disability, and inability to wear normal shoes
5. Nonoperative treatment
   a. Ponseti method of serial manipulation and long-leg casting, along with percutaneous Achilles tenotomy in most cases (well described in Clubfoot: Ponseti Management, LT Staheli, editor. www.Global-HELP.org monograph)
      i. It should be successful in at least 85% of idiopathic cases.
      ii. It should be successful in a smaller percentage of nonidiopathic (arthrogryposis, myelomeningocele) cases, but definitely worth the effort.

6. Operative indications
   a. Failure to achieve full deformity correction with non-operative treatment
7. Operative treatment with reference to the surgical techniques section of the book for each individual procedure
   a. Percutaneous tendo-Achilles tenotomy (**see Chapter 7**)—*perform this* when there is less than 10° of ankle dorsiflexion after the cavus, adductus, and varus have been fully corrected with serial casting in an infant or very young child
      i. This is a complete tenotomy, not a lengthening.
      ii. It should be performed when there is little (or no) expectation that a posterior ankle capsulotomy will be required, which is the assumption in most babies up to at least 2 years of age.
         • If a percutaneous tendo-Achilles tenotomy is concurrently converted to an open ankle capsulotomy, the gap in the tendon may not heal and remodel as well, and with as good preservation of excursion, as with percutaneous Achilles tenotomy alone.
      iii. If the need for a posterior capsulotomy is anticipated, an open tendo-Achilles lengthening should be performed. If a capsulotomy is then deemed unnecessary, there is no measureable disability from having performed a formal tendo-Achilles lengthening.
   b. Posterior release (**see Chapter 7**)—*perform this* in an older child in whom there is less than 10° of dorsiflexion after the cavus, adductus, and varus have been fully corrected with serial casting and in whom there is less than 10° of dorsiflexion after TAL
   c. À la carte partial-to-complete circumferential release (**see Chapter 7**)—*perform this* if there are residual cavus, adductus, and/or varus deformities in addition to an equinus deformity
      i. The McKay procedure is the surgical analog of the Ponseti method, in that it embraces the pathoanatomy ascribed to by Ponseti.

      ii. In *non*-idiopathic clubfoot (myelomeningocele, arthrogryposis), the tendons are released rather than lengthened, because of the very high recurrence rate in these feet.

Neglected Clubfoot

1. Definition—**Deformity**
   a. Untreated congenital equino-cavo-adducto-varus in an older child or adolescent (Figures 5-10 and 5-11)
2. Elucidation of the segmental deformities
   a. Forefoot—*pronated*
   b. Midfoot—*adducted*
   c. Hindfoot—*varus/inverted*
   d. Ankle—*plantar flexed (equinus)*
3. Imaging
   a. Standing AP and lateral of foot
   b. Standing AP and lateral of ankle
4. Natural history
   a. Persistence of deformity with pain, functional disability, and inability to wear normal shoes
5. Nonoperative treatment
   a. Ponseti method of serial manipulation and long-leg casting, along with percutaneous Achilles tenotomy in most cases (well described in Clubfoot: Ponseti Management, LT Staheli, editor. www.Global-HELP.org monograph), starting in children up to at least 5 to 6 years of age (and possibly older)
      i. Should be successful less often than when initiated in infants, with the rate of success inversely proportional to age at initiation
6. Operative indications
   a. Failure or age-inappropriateness of serial casting to correct one or more of the clubfoot segmental deformities
   b. Pain, shoe-fitting difficulties, dysfunction

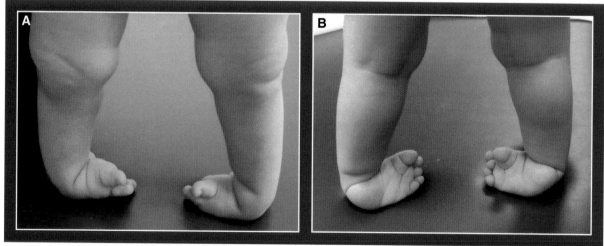

Figure 5-10. Untreated clubfeet in a 2-year-old boy who was adopted from a developing country by parents in the United States.

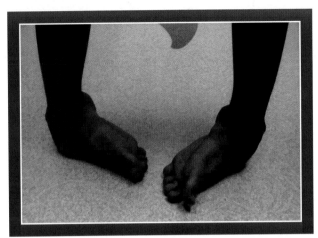

Figure 5-11. Neglected clubfeet in an 18-year-old immigrant to the United States. The natural history of clubfoot is clear: persistence of deformities, inability to wear shoes, ostracism, poverty, and eventual pain.

7. <u>Operative treatment</u> with reference to the surgical techniques section of the book for each individual procedure
   a. Percutaneous tendo-Achilles tenotomy (**see Chapter 7**)—*perform this* when there is less than 10° of ankle dorsiflexion after the cavus, adductus, and varus have been fully corrected with serial casting in a young child
      i. This is a complete tenotomy, not a lengthening.
      ii. It should be performed when there is little (or no) expectation that a posterior ankle capsulotomy will be required.
         • If a percutaneous tendo-Achilles tenotomy is concurrently converted to an open ankle capsulotomy, the gap in the tendon may not heal and remodel as well, and with as good preservation of excursion, as with percutaneous Achilles tenotomy alone.
      iii. If the need for a posterior capsulotomy is anticipated, an open tendo-Achilles lengthening should be performed. If a capsulotomy is then deemed unnecessary, there is no measureable disability from having performed a formal tendo-Achilles lengthening.
   b. Posterior release (**see Chapter 7**)—*perform this* if there is less than 10° of dorsiflexion after the cavus, adductus, and varus have been fully corrected with serial casting and the tendo-Achilles has been lengthened
   c. À la carte partial-to-complete circumferential release (**see Chapter 7**)—*perform this* if there are residual cavus, adductus, and/or varus deformities in addition to an equinus deformity
      i. The McKay procedure is the surgical analog of the Ponseti method, in that it embraces the pathoanatomy ascribed to by Ponseti.
      ii. In *non*-idiopathic clubfoot, the tendons are released rather than lengthened, because of the high recurrence rate in these feet.
   d. À la carte partial-to-complete circumferential release (**see Chapter 7**) *along with* one or more of the following

procedures—*perform one or more of these additional procedures* if there are residual cavus, adductus, and/or varus deformities in addition to an equinus deformity, *and* structural metatarsus adductus (MA), fixed hindfoot varus with a long lateral column of the foot, and/or muscle imbalance
      i. Medial column lengthening for structural MA
         • Medial cuneiform opening wedge osteotomy (**see Chapter 8**)
      ii. Lateral column shortening for structural MA (**see Management Principle #18, Chapter 4**)
         • Closing wedge osteotomy of the cuboid (**see Chapter 8**)
      iii. Lateral column shortening for resistant hindfoot varus/inversion with a long lateral column of the foot (**see Management Principle #18, Chapter 4**)
         • Calcaneocuboid resection/fusion (**see Chapter 8**)
         • Lichtblau resection of the anterior calcaneus (**see Chapter 8**)
         • Closing wedge osteotomy of the anterior calcaneus (**see Chapter 8**)
      iv. Posterior calcaneus lateral displacement osteotomy (**see Chapter 8**)
      v. Anterior tibialis tendon transfer to lateral (3rd) cuneiform (**see Chapter 7**)
   e. Triple arthrodesis (**see Chapter 8**)—*perform this* if there are *no* other options for correcting the deformities because of severity and/or rigidity, or because of existing degenerative arthritis of the subtalar joint (**see Management Principle #13, Chapter 4**)
   f. Gradual deformity correction with external fixation (not elucidated in this book)

Severe, Rigid, Resistant Arthrogrypotic Clubfoot in an Infant or Young Child

1. <u>Definition—**Deformity**</u>
   a. Severe, rigid, resistant congenital clubfoot in an infant with arthrogryposis (Figure 5-12)
   b. More flexible congenital clubfoot deformities in infants with arthrogryposis should be treated exactly like idiopathic congenital clubfoot (**see this chapter**).
2. <u>Elucidation of the segmental deformities</u>
   a. Forefoot—*pronated*
   b. Midfoot—*adducted*
   c. Hindfoot—*varus/inverted*
   d. Ankle—*plantar flexed (equinus)*
3. <u>Imaging</u>
   a. Maximum dorsiflexion/abduction/eversion AP and lateral of foot—indicated to:
      i. confirm residual deformities preoperatively after failing nonoperative treatment
4. <u>Natural history</u>
   a. Persistence of deformity with pain, functional disability, and inability to wear normal shoes